Praise for *Empowered Aging*

Empowered Aging is an authoritative and accessible guide to practicing yoga safely as you age. With crystal-clear instructions, as well as pointers to adapt and refine, this book is a must-have for practitioners and teachers alike. If you want to reap the wide-ranging benefits of yoga for vibrant and healthy aging—or if you teach people who do—get this book!

—**Barrie Risman**, author of *Evolving Your Yoga*

I've been studying yoga with Ellen Saltonstall since 2001 and credit what I've learned from her for being in good shape now at almost eighty. When I've taken a class with someone else over these twenty-two years, Ellen's teachings about anatomy and alignment have helped me stay safe and get the maximum benefit from each pose.

—**Joan Rothchild Hardin**, PhD, clinical psychologist in private practice

Ellen Saltonstall's statement at the beginning of *Empowered Aging* about yoga being "adaptable to different needs" is exactly how she teaches yoga for aging clients in this concise and informative book. I have studied with Ellen and in her book she pays just as much attention to detail and physical safety as she does in her studio. The poses she describes in the book have helped me move my osteoporosis numbers! I highly recommend it.

—**Joyce Cohen**, actor

Yoga has tremendous potential for helping us to maintain strength and balance as we age, both physically and emotionally. In *Empowered Aging*, longtime teacher Ellen Saltonstall makes these benefits accessible to people of all ages and ability levels, enabling you to begin with the yoga poses that are right for you, to modify your current practices as you experience age-related changes, and to progress at your own pace. This is truly empowering!

—**Nina Zolotow**, coauthor of *Yoga for Healthy Aging* and author of *Yoga for Times of Change*

If you are looking to enjoy the many age-defying benefits of yoga, *Empowered Aging* is for you! Ellen Saltonstall is a rare and gifted yoga teacher, who combines decades of study and teaching of yoga with a unique ability to make it enjoyable, inspiring and effective, no matter what your previous experience level is. Yoga is not a one-size-fits-all, and with the knowledge in this book, Ellen empowers the reader to make yoga their own and guides us brilliantly into that wonderful journey of transformation that is yoga.

—**Eva Norlyk Smith**, president of YogaUOnline

Ellen Saltonstall is one of New York City's and the world's best yoga teachers for students of all ages, abilities and experience. Her vast knowledge of yoga, movement, massage, anatomy and yoga therapeutics is on display in *Empowered Aging* for those new to yoga or for anyone looking for insight into body/mind integration and aging gracefully. Ellen's love for yoga and for the human spirit's potential shines through these pages. I've been practicing with Ellen for a decade. Her authoritative voice rings out in the text, and I am transported to her studio once again. What a blessing!

—**Louise Desjardins**, CYT Kripalu, Corepower and Restorative Yoga

As a meditation teacher, trainer and yogi for over forty years, I've had the opportunity to study with many outstanding, well-known teachers and, still, Ellen Saltonstall is the best! Her grasp of anatomy partnered with her skilled clear guidance is unparalleled. Stand up straight, walk briskly, and rush to get this new book. Plan to age in beauty, health and grace with Ellen's new book, *Empowered Aging.*

—**Kate Mitcheom**, MSN, CNM, RYT, certified senior teacher and trainer in MBSR and mindfulness programs

As a yoga teacher for twenty-five years, I had doubts that a book about yoga for beginners would be useful to me, but I was so wrong. Ellen Saltonstall had me from the first sentence—Yes! I do intend to stay strong and active as I age—and it kept me engaged all the way through. Ellen writes with a clarity and grace that appeals to beginners as well as longtime yogis. Her simply elegant explanations of complex subjects helps me help my students, and her approach to the sequencing of poses is brilliant.

—**Marianna Adams**, director of White Rock Yoga Dallas

I love this book! Although I have practiced yoga for over fifty years and taught for more than forty, I felt excited, like a beginner, reading this book. Ellen Saltonstall's writing is so informative, inspiring and fresh. One standout feature of *Empowered Aging* is its focus on joint and bone health. Ellen provides clear, detailed and encouraging guidance on proactively stimulating joint and bone health through yoga. Another gift of this book is its emphasis and encouragement to be more fully present, both during yoga practice as well as off the mat, as a way toward a better health span and self-care in daily life. *Empowered Aging* is a treasure and will be a permanent part of the yoga library at my school of yoga, as well as required reading for both our basic and advanced teacher training programs.

—**Karin Sprute-Francovich**, founder of Garden Street School of Yoga

What a great way for older folks to get started with yoga or to go deeper in their practice. The information and instructions in *Empowered Aging* are simple and clear, and yet they reflect Ellen's years of study, practice and experience with yoga. I can't wait to buy a copy for my older friends and relatives.

—**Jayendra Hanley**, curriculum development coordinator for Anusara Yoga and aging yoga practitioner and teacher

Hallelujah! How refreshing to find a yoga book geared toward people beyond the twenty-something or thirty-something age group. As someone with fifty years of yoga practice under my belt, I loved seeing each pose in *Empowered Aging* demonstrated by the author, a woman with greying hair and laugh lines. We may be in the second half of our lives, but we don't have to hang out in our rocking chairs.

Throughout the book, Ellen Saltonstall shares excellent advice to safely build bones and improve balance. *Empowered Aging* encourages everyone to find their own yoga practice, offering a variety of modifications. The layout is very clear and easy to follow, and I was pleased to see hand and wrist exercises, which I include in my bone health therapeutic workshops.

—**Deborah Charnes**, certified yoga therapist and author of *From the Boxing Ring to the Ashram*

Empowered Aging is an invitation and a guide to actively engage with one's health with wisdom and skill as one ages. Ellen Saltonstall's step-by-step guidance is clear and well-paced while emerging from a depth of knowledge and experience with yoga, anatomy and meditation. This book can build confidence in learning how to evoke resilience of the body, mind and heart. It offers a skillful way to befriend the changes, joys and challenges of aging with grace.

—**Florence Meleo Meyer**, director of teacher training at the Center for Mindfulness at UMass Memorial Health Center

In a world filled with advice on looking younger, along with drugs and devices laden with anti-aging promises, Ellen Saltonstall's new book offers real help and hope that there is much we can do to ameliorate the inevitable effects of having many birthdays. *Empowered Aging* is the product of nearly fifty years of study and practice by someone I trust completely. When my sister-in-law was suffering from chronic back pain, Ellen was the one who helped her beyond what the medical profession could offer. Today she is pain-free, thanks to the advice and instruction she received from Ellen. They say that aging is not for sissies. At sixty-five, I have to agree with that statement. Why not take these empowering steps toward feeling good in body and mind and fully enjoy this rich last chapter of our lives?

—**Desirée Rumbaugh**, certified yoga instructor and coauthor of *Fearless After Fifty*

Aging is a new season of our life, just as autumn is a new season after summer, and *Empowered Aging* is the perfect guide for this next season. In a simple and clear way, Ellen Saltonstall explains what happens in our body as we age and how yoga can support us in flowing through these changes. With its easy, detailed explanations and its insights to deepen our experience beyond the mat, it is a must-have book for all of us, both new or long-time yoga practitioners, juniors or seniors, students or teachers. Autumn can be as wonderful as summer, and we too can be incredibly colorful in the second part of our life!

—**Alessandra di Prampero**, Anusara Yoga teacher trainer

Ellen Saltonstall is a lifelong learner and a passionate and knowledgeable teacher. Her continued studies of anatomy have helped her craft wonderful techniques for her students. She never stops questioning how the body, mind and spirit can work best together. *Empowered Aging* promises to be a must-read for anyone who is interested in yoga and aging.

—**Dr. Christine Benner**, DC, LAc, MSHAPI, CSCP

My favorite line in Ellen Saltonstall's book is, "Remember, how you do the poses is more important than which poses you do." *Empowered Aging* offers yoga as a body/mind skill accessible to anyone at any age, and any level of ability. In her book, Ellen provides expert advice on how to protect your body when doing poses along with excellent suggestions for using props and practical variations for teaching seniors. With her focus on healthy aging, balance and the health of your joints, muscles and bones, she has provided a practical method to bring the ageless wisdom of yoga into our modern world. She reminds readers to listen to their bodies and explore how the pose or movement feels for them in order to vary it according to their personal needs and stage of life. There is something for everyone on the yoga path in this book.

—Beth Gibbs, author of *Enlighten Up!*

I highly recommend *Empowered Aging* and think the focus on the internal sensations and awareness of the body is especially important and needed. The yoga sequences are excellent and are appropriate for those with osteopenia and mild osteoporosis.

—Deirdre Finn, founder of Finn Physical Therapy

In *Empowered Aging*, Ellen Saltonstall has given you a handy set of tools in the form of movement sequences that you can easily access with her simple, clear instructions and no-nonsense information. Her positive reframing of aging will inspire you to take matters into your own hands and then reap the benefits!

—Gabriella Barnstone, founder of Scoliosis Conditioning

EMPOWERED AGING

Other books by Ellen Saltonstall
   Yoga for Arthritis
   Yoga for Osteoporosis
   Anatomy and Yoga
   The Bodymind Ballwork Method

EMPOWERED AGING

*Everyday Yoga Practices
for Bone Health,
Strength and
Balance*

ELLEN
SALTONSTALL

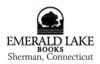

EMERALD LAKE
BOOKS
Sherman, Connecticut

Empowered Aging: Everyday Yoga Practices for Bone Health, Strength and Balance

Copyright © 2024 Ellen Saltonstall

Cover illustration © 2024 by Mark Gerber

Photo credits: Max Saltonstall, Josef Kushner and Lynn Saltonstall

Interior illustrations © 2024 by Emily Ciosek

Library of Congress Cataloging-in-Publication Data

Names: Saltonstall, Ellen, author.

Title: Empowered aging : everyday yoga practices for bone health, strength and balance / by Ellen Saltonstall.

Description: Sherman : Emerald Lake Books, [2024] | Includes bibliographical references and index.

Identifiers: LCCN 2023031143 (print) | LCCN 2023031144 (ebook) | ISBN 9781945847745 (paperback) | ISBN 9781945847752 (epub)

Subjects: LCSH: Yoga--Health aspect. | Yoga--Therapeutic use. | Bones--Diseases--Prevention.

Classification: LCC RA781.7 .S244 2024 (print) | LCC RA781.7 (ebook) | DDC 613.7/046--dc23/eng/20230719

LC record available at https://lccn.loc.gov/2023031143

LC ebook record available at https://lccn.loc.gov/2023031144

Books published by Emerald Lake Books may be ordered through your favorite booksellers or by visiting emeraldlakebooks.com.

To my teachers, students, colleagues and readers
who are carrying the traditions of yoga forward
for the benefit of all.

Table of Contents

Preface

Do you intend to remain strong and active throughout your life? If you have physical limitations, exercise can feel risky, but if you proceed carefully with appropriate guidance, you can do it safely, starting from exactly where you are right now.

Perhaps your friends, family or healthcare practitioners have suggested that you try yoga, or perhaps you have lapsed and are ready to return. This book offers you a carefully created yoga program that will help you build strength and enjoy a new vitality throughout your elder years.

How am I qualified to guide you on this journey? I encountered yoga in my midtwenties through my spiritual community, first as meditation and then as a physical practice. My work at that time involved a combination of modern dance and massage therapy. I have always had a fascination with—and reverence for—the human body: how it works, how we take care of it, and how we express ourselves through it. With hatha yoga, I found a physical practice that combined my spiritual quest with my enjoyment of movement.

Once my three children were grown, I turned my focus more to the therapeutic aspects of yoga and how it can help people of all ages to live fully. Through my teaching and studies with master teachers, I have developed methodologies to help people with their aches and pains, as well as their resistance to exercise. Giving people confidence and information to implement the practice that meets their needs has been my mission.

Arthritis and osteoporosis are conditions that develop slowly over time and generally affect people in their fifties and above.

With arthritis, the inner lining of our joints gradually wears down, creating uneven surfaces and extra bone growth, along with pain and restricted movement. If you have arthritis, you may be hesitant to exercise for fear of pain. Osteoporosis is a thinning of the bone's inner structure, potentially leading to a fracture. With osteoporosis, you may find yourself fearful of doing anything that increases the risk of fracturing a bone.

In teaching yoga and Bodymind Ballwork for over forty-five years, I have seen repeatedly that those fears can be overcome and we can maintain a healthy, active lifestyle, even if there are restrictions. Yoga is the perfect methodology to counter aging because it's adaptable to different needs. It is a living tradition with deep roots in the past but also constantly evolving along with modern life.

I've taught many workshops on yoga for osteoporosis, and I continue to develop my programs and learn from my students. Yoga studios in Europe and around the United States have invited me to teach this material to the public and in teacher training programs.

This book has evolved from many of my handouts, courses and webinars with the goal of offering a reference guide for anyone who would like to continue this marvelous practice on their own.

Students often tell me:

> *I'm afraid of doing yoga because I am not flexible and I might hurt myself.*

I understand that caution. But in working with thousands of students, I've seen that, with reliable information, you can get beyond that fear to begin a renewed connection with your body—one that enlivens your everyday life. Don't let your previous lack of exercise stop you from starting fresh!

Perhaps you are thinking that yoga is all about touching your toes or wrapping your arms and legs into extreme positions? That's the media version. The real-life version invites you to start wherever you are and work intelligently from there, with many choices to be made along the way. Yoga offers a path for self-understanding and transformational growth that welcomes you at any stage of your life, despite the health challenges you may have. You learn to love and respect your body with all its quirkiness and limitations. What you need is reliable information and compassionate guidance from a qualified teacher, which is what I provide here.

So, this book is for you if you:

- want a user-friendly entry into the practice of yoga.
- want to age gracefully and remain active.
- have osteopenia or osteoporosis.
- would benefit from a guide to develop a home practice.
- teach yoga, especially for seniors.

If you already have a regular yoga practice, I hope you will gain some new insights and variations to add to your repertoire. If you are a teacher, I hope this book will enrich what you have to offer to your students.

How to Use This Book

I developed the methodology outlined in *Empowered Aging* specifically for those with osteopenia, osteoporosis or other age-related health challenges, but what I teach here is suitable for anyone who wants a practice that is safe and empowering. My intent is to help you learn, pursue and perhaps teach physical yoga in a way that is beneficial as aging becomes more evident. For each pose, I provide a description and illustrations, indicating its benefits and how to adapt it to your individual needs.

This book is intended to be a companion on your path of learning. Whether you are a beginner or an experienced yoga practitioner, my detailed instructions will help you learn about your body and make smart choices in how you use it—in everyday activities and while you exercise.

The first chapters provide an overview of what yoga is and what it can do for you, with answers to some common questions asked by my potential students. Then I outline the normal process of aging, noting important considerations and helpful tips that apply to exercising in our senior years.

Before getting into the actual poses, it's important to understand some of the terms that are used in the instructions. So I've provided a lexicon that defines key words and phrases to make it easy for you to interpret the pose directions.

The subsequent chapters contain the instructions for the poses and are organized like a menu—appetizers, main dishes, side dishes, desserts—covering recommended warm-ups, strengthening techniques, chair practices, and cool-down routines. I encourage you to choose options from each menu to create a practice that works for you.

In this book, I refer to the poses as they are commonly known in English, followed by the commonly accepted Sanskrit name where appropriate. (Some poses are variations on the classic pose of that name.) You may find if you attend a class in person that some instructors will use the Sanskrit name and others won't, and their pronunciations may vary. While many poses were identified in ancient Indian texts thousands of years ago, others have been added as the practice evolved. The names refer to various things, including body positions, animals, aspects of nature, or heroes and deities from Indian mythology, which can evoke subtleties for your practice as you dig deeper into the traditions of yoga. Don't worry if you can't pronounce the Sanskrit!

A quick visual reference in the margin identifies the practices that are best for improving bone health, strength or balance. I also share some of the finer points for each pose that will enable you to refine your technique as you become more familiar with it. This is followed by instructions for doing the pose and then reflection questions that will help make the practice more personal.

I have provided a list of suggested sequences just before the pose chapters, and my hope is that you will be able to design your own plan as you become familiar with all the options available to you.

Each chapter has a specific focus with multiple options to choose from. While each pose may have lengthy instructions, once you practice them a few times, you will only need to read the instructions for review.

To do all the poses in this book would take more than two hours, but that's not necessary. I suggest that you practice all the elements from each chapter a few times, then choose certain

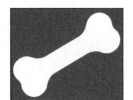

Bone Health

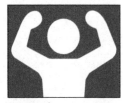

Strength

Balance

ones to work with for a week or two, especially if they target an aging issue you hope to improve. After that, change it up for variety and fun.

If you'd like to dive deeper, I've included additional resources in the recommended reading that are useful for further study.

I hope that this book will not only guide you on your path of learning, but inspire you to remain curious to see what you'll discover on the way. The practice reveals its benefits as we do it. It's one thing to read about yoga, but it's a whole other thing to do it regularly and authentically explore how it can transform your life as you improve your bone health, strength and balance.

Chapter 1. Yoga Is for Everyone

Yoga is a practice for everyone—from children to the elderly and those in between. With yoga, we become more centered as we build and maintain healthy muscles. Our bones strengthen, and we have improved breathing, better coordination and balance—all things that will help us live a full life. Physical and mental empowerment both sustain us as we age. Even if chronic medical conditions present some limitations, yoga can be adapted for any level of fitness. It's not one size fits all, and you don't have to stand on your head or fold into a pretzel. Your yoga practice can be customized by you, for you.

With the increasing awareness of yoga in Western culture, you might think that yoga is all about physical training. But in addition to those benefits, yoga can show you a deeper part of yourself in which you are emotionally uplifted, strong in your mind and heart, grounded and at peace. This can come from the physical practice alone, but I find that many students feel inspired to try the other aspects of yoga, such as pranayama (breathing exercises) and meditation.

The style of yoga I teach originates with my studies of Iyengar yoga and Anusara yoga, both of which are focused on precise alignment of the body. My style provides a pathway to self-understanding through physical postures, breathing and meditation. While this book only covers the physical poses I teach, they can be added to any style of yoga you may already practice.

Yoga offers the kind of exercise you can maintain for your entire life. As Steven Covey, author of *The Seven Habits of Highly Effective People* (Simon and Schuster, 1989), puts it:

> *Most of us think we don't have enough time to exercise. What a distorted paradigm! We don't have time not to. (p. 289)*

From my decades of work in the fields of body awareness and fitness, my mission with this book is to give you confidence—confidence to start a practice if you're new to yoga, confidence to adapt your practice as you feel the effects of aging, and confidence to progress at your own pace.

You may have some other specific questions or concerns holding you back from adding yoga to your wellness practices, especially if you have a diagnosis of osteoporosis or osteopenia. Here are some of the most common questions I've heard from students who are considering studying with me.

1. **Why is this program of yoga poses especially good for those with osteoporosis?**

   I will address this question in more detail on page 14, but in brief, here are some benefits that can be attained through yoga.
   - You will learn poses that specifically help you develop good balance, thereby preventing falls.
   - You will learn your optimum alignment so you can get the most out of your practice while protecting your joints.
   - You will gain muscle strength, which is essential for an active life.
   - You will learn a variety of positions that give ample stimulation to the bones to strengthen them.
   - You can adapt the poses to any level of fitness and yoga experience. There are variations to most poses that allow you to progress at your own pace.
   - Most of all, you will gain confidence to move more, and that is beneficial for general vitality.

2. **Why do I need yoga if I already go to the gym and play sports?**

   Sports and gym workouts are beneficial for general fitness and fun, especially when we are young. Yoga offers an exercise regimen that can be adapted as you age. You can practice yoga as a warm-up or cool-down along with those other pursuits. You'll be building strength, flexibility and self-awareness in a different way. My style of yoga emphasizes optimal alignment and mindfulness, as well as the connection to a deeper personal transformation. It will enhance whatever other physical practices you do. As I discuss later, the recommendations in this book are geared toward strengthening muscles and bones.

3. **What if it hurts when I try to do yoga?**

   Pain is a warning signal, telling you to pay attention. It's part of our arsenal of survival mechanisms. It can be chronic or acute, and it urges us to make changes.

   But pain is also subjective, influenced by the circumstances and context. We each have a different level of tolerance for pain. Negative expectations are known to amplify pain. Sometimes when we feel a strong sensation, we fear it is a sign of injury or damage to the body. While that might be true, more often in yoga, the strong sensations are from learning a new physical skill or doing something familiar, but in a new way that creates more demand. Hurt and harm are not the same.

   You can minimize the chance of pain or injury by making the commitment to practice carefully with good warm-ups. Find the right balance between doing too much and doing too little. If the discomfort from your practice is consistent or worsening, consult a qualified yoga teacher or healthcare professional.

4. **How often should I practice and for how long?**

   I recommend doing yoga daily, whether it's twenty minutes or more. But you need to think about your goals and the practicalities of your life. What are you willing to commit to? When is the best time of day for you? What are your goals? That's the challenge of an independent practice: having the clarity of purpose and the discipline to do it! A significant part of your yoga experience is making choices based on what's most helpful for you. It may be easier to work with a teacher who creates the structure for you. Do that as often as you can. Another possibility is to enjoy yoga with one or two friends for mutual support and companionship. But however you choose to structure your practice, you must do it regularly to reap the benefits.

5. **How do I decide what poses to do and in what order?**

You may feel unsure of what to do in your mind, but your body will tell you. Refer to my suggestions on page xxiii about how to use this book. Once you've tried everything at least once, design a sequence that feels good and addresses your goals. Be sure to include some warm-ups, gentle poses, and a few challenging ones. Practice that for a week or two, and then add in more elements as you feel ready. I offer some suggested sequences on page 41.

6. **I don't have yoga props. Can I still give yoga a try?**

Yes, you can do many of the yoga practices in this book with just a floor, chair and wall. Each pose description includes which props are recommended. You can also find a list of suitable substitutes on page 37.

7. **I've been practicing yoga for thirty years, and I love it. Do I have to change what I'm doing if I have a diagnosis of osteopenia or osteoporosis?**

Hopefully, your favorite poses are safe for you. Remember, how you do the pose is just as important as which pose you do. If your practice has been more relaxed and stretchy, I recommend focusing more on building strength. If your practice is vigorous, take the precautions listed in the next answer. If you consider your practice to be moderate (neither too gentle nor too strenuous), congratulations! That's the safest route to take. We want to challenge ourselves while remaining safe, and finding that delicate balance is a yogic skill in itself!

8. **What are some common yoga practices I should avoid if I have reduced bone density?**

   Not all yoga poses are safe to do when your bones are more brittle. Consider avoiding:
   - fast sun salutations, especially with jumps.
   - standing or seated forward bends with both legs straight and close together, especially curling down into the pose one vertebra at a time.
   - twists with a curved spine or forceful use of your arms.
   - inversions without support nearby.

To build confidence, you need good information. In this book, you'll find detailed instructions for optimal alignment and beneficial actions, and the information you need to create a safe practice you will enjoy and pursue regularly. The familiar adage "use it or lose it" is so true when it comes to our bodies and minds.

But before we explore the poses, let's look at how yoga came to the West from India and how its traditions from ancient times have continued and evolved over the years. Each of us can partake in the richness of the tradition, regardless of our current strength or flexibility, and creatively add a personal touch to it.

Chapter 2. Making Yoga Your Own

The practices of yoga originated in India thousands of years ago. But it wasn't until the late nineteenth and mid-twentieth centuries that knowledge of this ancient tradition began to spread. Around that time, some teachers came from India to America, including Swami Vivekananda, who spoke at the World Parliament of Religions in Chicago in 1893. Gradually, Americans began traveling to India to learn from yogis there, then returned home to spread the word.

By the 1970s, yoga had become a cultural phenomenon in America. As of 2023, 36 million people in America (one in nine) practice some form of yoga. More than half of those practicing yoga are in their fifties or older.[1]

From those ancient roots and in the process of teacher-to-student transmission, many pathways of yoga have emerged, all in the service of inner transformation and growth. In case you think yoga is only about physical postures and stretching, here's a short list of the main historical branches of yoga practice.

- Hatha yoga: the path of physical postures (asana) and breathing exercises (pranayama)
- Bhakti yoga: the path of devotion to one's chosen deity
- Karma yoga: the path of compassionate service to community
- Jnana yoga: the path of knowledge and studying scriptures
- Raja yoga: the path of meditation

---

1   Jeong, Soomi. "Yoga Facts, Industry Statistics," Yogi Times, September 11, 2023. ellensaltonstall.com/trends.

As you can see from this list, the physical practice of hatha yoga is only one branch of a vast tree. But you don't need to confine yourself to just one yoga path. You can combine the practices of the various branches. For instance, you can perform the physical practices, offer service, and meditate to come up with a blend that's completely yours.

Within the realm of hatha yoga, many lineages of teachers and their students have put their stamp on how the yoga practice is done. Each style combines some aspects of physical, mental and spiritual health with its own emphasis. But each tradition recognizes and promotes these benefits in some way. For example:

- greater self-understanding and equanimity
- improved breathing
- physical fitness, including both strength and flexibility
- lower risk of injury as compared to other fitness practices
- pain relief
- stress relief and mental clarity
- improvement of sleep and mood

For more information about yoga traditions, I recommend these sources:

Feuerstein, Georg. *The Yoga Tradition: Its History, Literature, Philosophy and Practice* (Chino Valley, AZ: Hohm Press, 2001).

Rakicevic, Mira. "31 Amazing Yoga Statistics," Disturb Me Not, January 12, 2022. ellensaltonstall.com/disturbmenot.

Singleton, Mark. *Yoga Body: The Origins of Modern Postural Practice* (Oxford: Oxford University Press, 2010).

Master yoga teacher B. K. S. Iyengar said:

> *The study of asana is not about mastering posture. It's about using posture to understand and transform yourself.*

One of my teachers, Mary Dunn, taught her own version of this.

> *First you learn about the poses, and then you learn about yourself in the poses.*

Each committed practitioner of yoga eventually branches beyond the techniques they've learned to make yoga their own.

I have pondered this a lot over my many decades of practice. What are we really practicing? Are we just making shapes? Stretching? Getting a spiritual workout? Embodying ancient wisdom?

While my approach to teaching yoga rests on traditions that are thousands of years old and my thoughts have been greatly influenced by my teachers, at a certain point, I wanted to distill my personal approach into a paradigm. It can be summarized as "ABC," which stands for: **a**wareness, the **b**alance of opposites, and **c**reative expression.

I've provided a brief overview of my personal paradigm below. If you're interested in exploring it more, you can find an expanded explanation at ellensaltonstall.com/abcs.

A for Awareness

In yoga, the practice of awareness can take many forms. The first and most important step is to become aware of yourself in the present moment.

Here are some questions that might trigger your awareness:

- Can you feel the movement of your breath?
- What other body sensations are you aware of?
- Do you have physical limitations, such as osteoarthritis or recent injuries, that will influence your yoga practice?
- What is your state of being, your energetic presence right now?
- Do you feel focused? Distracted? Tired? Energized? Sad? Content? Calm? Curious? Anything else?

Keep in mind, awareness is separate from analysis and judgment! Try to let all sensations and thoughts register without categorizing or rating them. Instead, be a compassionate witness to your moment to moment experience of being alive.

B for the Balance of Opposites

One of my teachers once said, "There are only two mistakes people make in yoga: working too hard or not working hard enough." Despite the humor in this statement, it is true for any kind of exercise. We can be so enthusiastic that we overdo our workouts and try to accomplish too much too soon. On the other side of the spectrum, you might hear this common yoga instruction: "Do only what's comfortable for you," which could mean we never challenge ourselves to learn something new or to work past perceived limitations.

The third way is to find the middle path between the two extremes—in this case, between effort and ease. Learn how to put enough energy into your practice to build both strength and flexibility, but also take care not to overdo it.

As I developed my ABC paradigm, I realized that this idea of finding the middle way between two apparent opposites can be explored in many intriguing ways. In the body, some of the opposites we can consider include the structural opposites of front and back, left and right, top and bottom, extremities and center.

Here are a few examples of finding the place of balance in the middle, between awareness and actions that may seem contradictory at first. But when these two facets are combined, they create a healthy pose.

1. **Root to Rise.** Every yoga pose has a base that supports our weight and touches the floor, whether it is in the feet, hands, pelvis, shoulders or some other part of the body. We can simultaneously reach down into that base ("root") and lift up and away from it ("rise"). The more we connect downward to the base, the more we can elongate upward. For instance, in a standing pose, the pelvis and legs root into the earth, while the torso and spine rise. We feel solidly grounded and yet expanded and light simultaneously.

2. **Front and Back.** When working on a yoga pose, we may notice sensations in either the front or back of our body more, based on where our attention is needed and more muscular work is happening. For example, in a back-bending pose, we can feel muscles contracting to create the arched shape of the spine. If we add another action of expanding the front, the pose becomes more complete, safe and enjoyable.

3. **Stability and Mobility.** Consider this: Is your body type muscular and possibly stiff and tight? If so, you might start doing yoga to become more flexible. Or are you more flexible, with easily bendable joints and stretchy muscles? In that case, yoga can help you to build strength.

In addition to how we train, each of us has characteristic types of connective tissue and muscles that will determine whether our body is looser and more flexible or tighter and more compact. During yoga, we work to bring balance to the tissues of the body and to the pose itself. We can pull into our center, creating stability. But we can also send energy from the center of the body out to the periphery, creating expansion. I call this the "stabilizing and expanding energies," and it is a central element in the techniques presented in this book. The invisible, vibrant power created by this balance of opposite energies makes the poses come alive.

To experience these complementary energies, here's a short exercise.

    a. Start with your arms extending to the sides while sitting or standing.

    b. With your arm muscles firmly contracting, imagine pulling your arms into the shoulder sockets.

    c. Squeeze your shoulder blades together. Feel the stability that gives to your joints, supported by the muscles and connective tissues.

    d. Add another equal current of energy that extends from your spine all the way to your fingertips, literally expanding your reach.

With those two opposites balanced, you'll have tremendous strength while retaining mobility.

C for Creative Expression

Often, people go to an exercise class and do what they're told without investigating things for themselves. Keep in mind that this practice is for you, and you have a role in creating it. I invite you to follow my instructions carefully, but also to remember that each of us is unique. So don't approach yoga in a mechanical way, without introspection. Explore the poses and how they feel to you. Even though some aspects of yoga are centuries old, we create a new experience each time we go onto the mat.

I recommend modifying postures to adapt to your needs and desires while remaining safe. Once you know the basics of a pose, play with it. Make a standing pose into more of a backbend, a twist or a forward bend. Find variations that stretch you in a new way. Use props to experiment with challenging balance postures. Connect the sequences in creative ways. Use music to find a refreshing rhythm in your body. Try doing your poses outdoors on a hillside.

Shake things up, be creative, and try things "out of the box." It's a good way to keep the practice fresh and alive. Yoga can offer so much more than just flexibility of the body. As you make your way through this book, you will be participating in time-honored practices while learning to make them your own.

But before we explore the poses, let's look first at the aging process and how it affects our muscles, bones and balance.

Chapter 3. **The Effects of Aging on the Body**

Increasing numbers of people are exploring yoga as a safe way to maintain their health when the signs of aging start to develop. Perhaps you are one of those! Many medical professionals recommend yoga to their patients for both physical and mental health issues, especially chronic pain and anxiety. We can't avoid aging, but we can prevent or slow down some of the health issues that develop in our later years. Research shows that it really works![2]

Well-being is more than just the absence of disease. With yoga, we can reduce many symptoms while also experiencing greater vitality with more mental equanimity, peace of mind and heart, and energy for life. We are fertilizing the soil of the body/mind garden and enjoying the harvest.

Here are some of the common changes that we might expect as we age.

- Less acuity in the nervous system, which could manifest as diminished sensory and motor efficiency, slower response time, and reduced coordination, as well as sparking cognitive decline
- Reduced awareness of the body in motion
- Poor balance, resulting from all the above
- Blood pressure deviations from normal levels
- Reduced circulatory efficiency and elasticity of blood vessels

---

2   The US National Library of Medicine's PubMed lists over 26K studies related to the health benefits of yoga. ncbi.nlm.nih.gov/pmc/?term=yoga.

- Loss of muscle strength (called "sarcopenia")[3]
- Stiffening of the connective tissues
- Loss of bone density
- Degeneration of joints due to wear and tear (osteoarthritis),[4] creating pain, followed by a downward spiral of diminished movement

For more information about studies that have evaluated the health benefits of yoga, I recommend these sources:

Madhivanan, Purnima, et al. "Yoga for Healthy Aging: Science or Hype?" *Advanced Geriatric Medical Research*, 3 (3), 2021. doi: 10.20900/agmr20210016.

McCall, Timothy. *Yoga as Medicine* (Random House, 2007).

Singh, Sat Bir, Lorenzo Cohen, Timothy McCall, and Shirley Telles, eds. *The Principles and Practice of Yoga in Health Care* (Handspring Publishing, 2016).

Despite all these potential changes, there are many things you can do to be empowered in the aging process. Yoga practice helps us develop better coordination, improving our daily life considerably. As we age, our bones become more brittle, and the danger of fracturing a bone if we fall increases. However, one of the many benefits of yoga is better balance, making us less likely to fall.

Osteoporosis

Bones are totally alive. They grow and develop through the first several decades of life. To remain strong, bones need exercise (and a good diet). However, just like any part of the human body, the passage of time leads to structural changes in bones.

Osteoporosis is a condition in which the bones gradually lose their normal density, becoming more fragile and susceptible to fractures. Our bones are strongest in our twenties and thirties, then begin to lose strength in our forties and fifties.

The term "osteopenia" is used to describe a precondition of osteoporosis, in which bones have lost some density but not to the extent that defines osteoporosis. If you have that diagnosis, it's a warning.

---

3 Studies show a connection between muscle loss and cognitive decline, according to an article by Gunner De Winter called "Aging and the Interplay Between Losing Muscle and Cognitive Function." (October 28, 2022.) ellensaltonstall.com/losingmuscle.

4 For more information about yoga for osteoarthritis, see my earlier book called *Yoga for Arthritis*, coauthored with Dr. Loren Fishman (W.W. Norton & Company, 2008).

Why heed that warning? If your pelvic bone or spinal vertebra or wrist is fractured, you may have to reduce your activities, which causes other progressive health challenges like muscle weakness, depression and social isolation.

Osteoporosis is not life-threatening, but the complications from osteoporotic fractures may cause a drastically reduced lifestyle.

Here are some questions I often hear about osteoporosis.

How common is osteoporosis? Are men at risk as much as women?

According to the Bone Health and Osteoporosis Foundation, osteoporosis and osteopenia is diagnosed in women and men of all races and ethnic groups, affecting about 54 million adults in the US as of 2023. For people over the age of fifty, an estimated one in two women and one in four men will have an osteoporosis-related fracture in their lifetime.[5] Although older men do develop low bone density, women are more at risk because they begin with less bone mass, and they lose it at a faster rate as they age because of hormonal changes associated with menopause. Osteoporosis is most common in non-Hispanic White women and Asian women, whereas African American and Hispanic women have a lower risk.[6]

How is osteoporosis diagnosed?

Often, people have no symptoms until they fall and fracture a bone. For those over sixty-five (or over fifty with specific risk factors), healthcare professionals recommend a test to determine the thickness of the bone and therefore its resistance to fracture. With a baseline measurement as a starting point, you can track changes if they occur.

A dual energy x-ray absorptiometry (DEXA) scan is the test used to diagnose osteoporosis. According to an established scale, your score on this scan tells whether you have normal density, osteopenia or osteoporosis.

Very low levels of x-rays are sent through the bone to determine how much of that signal is absorbed and how much passes

---

5   "Bone Health Basics: Get the Facts," Bone Health and Osteoporosis Foundation. Accessed August 14, 2023. ellensaltonstall.com/bonehealth.
6   "Osteoporosis," National Institute of Arthritis and Musculoskeletal and Skin Diseases, December 2022. ellensaltonstall.com/osteoporosis.

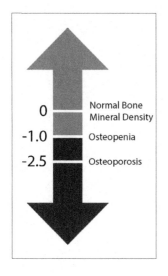

through. This testing is done on the bones that fracture the most commonly: the lumbar vertebrae and parts of the pelvis and femur.

The score from the DEXA scan tells you how much your density varies from that of the average healthy thirty-year-old adult (the T-score), and how much your density varies from other people of your age, weight and height (the Z-score). These scores are computed by a complex formula.

A T-score of -1 to -2.5 indicates a diagnosis of osteopenia, which is an early stage of bone thinning, while one of -2.5 or below indicates a diagnosis of osteoporosis. That means that you have thinner bones than 99 percent of thirty-year-old adults at the peak of their bone strength.

It's interesting to note that the machines used to measure bone density were developed by the same company that produced the first drugs to treat the condition.[7] Marketing motivations are a part of our modern culture, in medicine as in any other industry. That said, the DEXA scan is an effective and trusted screening tool for predicting fractures from low bone density.

What's actually happening inside a normal bone?

Bone cells are constantly being remodeled by cells called "osteo-blasts" and "osteoclasts." Osteoblasts secrete the raw mate-

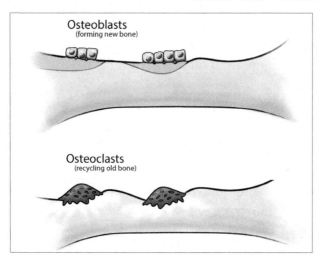

rials for new bone, which then harden. This process is influenced by thyroid and parathyroid hormones as well as growth hormones, estrogen and progesterone.

Just as the osteoblasts are making new bone, the osteoclasts are destroying old bone and clearing away debris; a process called "resorption." Protein and minerals are recycled back into the bloodstream.

During the third and fourth decades of life, the balance between building and recycling tips in favor of the osteoclasts

---

7   Alix Spiegel, "How a Bone Disease Grew to Fit a Prescription," All Things Considered, NPR, December 21, 2009. ellensaltonstall.com/prescription.

and more bone is destroyed than created, causing bones to become weaker.

The balance between these two is the elusive part. We don't really know what makes the osteoclasts take over and weaken bones as osteoporosis develops.

Are there other factors besides bone density that affect bone strength and risk of fracture?

Bone density or thickness is only one factor that's relevant in terms of the risk of fracture. What's not measured in the DEXA scan is the internal structure of the bone or a person's balance, strength, flexibility and lifestyle. How susceptible to falling are they? Are they sedentary or are they a mountain climber, stunt double, or elite athlete?

New studies are in place to develop testing with magnetic resonance imaging (MRI) that will assess the quality of the internal structure and how well it provides strength to the inside of the bone. Having this MRI assessment could lead you to make decisions regarding whether and how to improve your bone quality, for instance, by challenging your bones more in your exercise routines and daily life.

Most bones have two basic parts: cortical (on the outside) and trabecular (on the inside). Cortical bone, also called "compact bone," is quite solid and accounts for 60 percent of a bone's strength. The trabecular bone has a lattice-like structure. There is significant variation between individuals in how this inner lattice work is arranged, which, of course, determines the strength and quality of the bone. Tests to measure this are now in development.

Healthy Bone

Thinning Bone

Cortical Bone

Trabecular Bone

What will your doctor recommend if you receive a diagnosis of osteoporosis?

The short answer is: medications, weight-bearing exercise, and calcium and vitamin D supplements. There are several types of medications that regulate the balance of bone creation and resorption. Each has side effects, which you should discuss with your physician.

A common medical recommendation for exercise is to do impact exercises, like jogging, which will build the leg bones and boost cardiovascular health. People are also told to be extra careful to avoid falling. But what if they can't do conventional exercise because of other health issues, like arthritic knees or hips? They have a dilemma—they are told they need one kind of exercise to build bone strength, but another one for joint safety.

Yoga is well suited to address both conditions.

Studies have shown that calcium and vitamin D will help to supply the raw material needed for bone growth, but without exercise, bone strength is still lost. So it's not just a matter of incorporating supplements or exercise into your life. Both are necessary.

Why is prevention the best approach?

Even though some bone loss is inevitable with aging, the best antidote to osteoporosis is prevention—to build bone mass before the age of thirty. It's like putting money in the bank, so once the normal thinning happens, there's enough to spare.

Bone loss is a gradual process for everyone between thirty and sixty-five, but after that, it speeds up. The challenge is to find a way to counter the natural process that's going to happen. Studies have shown that the best way to build bone mass is through exercise.

How does exercise help bones to stay strong?

This bears repeating: bones are alive. They grow when they are exposed to stress, which can be either compression stress or tensile stress. Compression stress is related to gravity. When we are standing, walking, running, dancing or doing sports or yoga, the bones are undergoing compression stress from gravity. Tensile stress occurs when the muscles pull on the bones during any activity, especially when parts of the body move away from the midline. Both compression and tensile stress help keep the bones strong.

A doctor and anatomist named Julius Wolff discovered the effect of stress on the bones in the late 1800s. He developed what's known as "Wolff's Law," which states that the design and inner structure of bone follow the lines of force to which that bone is subjected. There is an electric charge generated in the bone cells in response to mechanical pressure, and that charge tells the osteoblasts to build more bone where more strength is needed.

Why is yoga a good way to exercise for those with decreased bone density?

Most students coming to yoga classes with osteoporosis are over fifty, and many will also have some arthritis or other joint difficulties. They are looking for a way to exercise that will stimulate their bones, yet not jar their joints. Yoga can provide compressive stress while in a standing position and also tensile stress when parts of the body are held off-center by the muscles. Since most yoga poses involve moving and holding the body in this way, such as doing side angle pose and chair pose, there is always tensile stress on the pelvic and spinal bones. Much of the yoga practice includes both types of stress, without the impact that might damage arthritic joints.

This is why yoga is so good for bone stimulation: we use such diverse positions that the bones receive a wide variety of pressure and stimulation for growth. I recommend holding the poses for fifteen to thirty seconds, giving time for your bones and soft tissue to receive the benefits of the stimulation. We can also hold yoga poses for longer than this, which magnifies their bone-building effects.

Yoga has the added advantage of being very adaptable to different ages and levels of ability. Props can be used to help stiffer students, and many poses develop balancing skills.

Are there contraindicated yoga poses?

Yes, there are yoga poses that may be contraindicated for those with low bone density. The strongest caution concerns any pose that involves bending forward or transitioning quickly into that position.

For people with weaker bones, bending forward could increase the risk of fracture (especially in the mid and lower back) if it's done with force, speed and a rounded spine, such as in sit-ups.

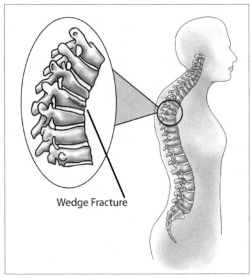

Wedge Fracture

In this case, the front of the vertebrae receives excessive pressure, which can eventually cause any single vertebra in that area to collapse into what's called a "wedge fracture." With less support in the spine because of this fracture, one's basic posture becomes stooped forward, creating the precondition for another fracture.

In addition, bending forward increases the risk of putting excess pressure on the spinal discs, which are cushions between the vertebrae that change shape as you move. When a fracture exists, the disc could be pushed to the back, where it might bulge and put pressure on the spinal nerves.

All yoga poses have the potential to strengthen the hip and spinal muscles, creating an important protection from fracture. In "Chapter 4. Before You Begin" on page 33, I provide a list of general cautions and specific guidance for achieving this goal.

Why is yoga particularly beneficial if you have a diagnosis of osteopenia or osteoporosis?

- Yoga is adaptable to any level of fitness or health and any age.
- Yoga practice improves body awareness.
- Yoga builds both strength and flexibility.
- Yoga improves your posture and breathing.
- Yoga can be practiced slowly and carefully to reduce the chances of falling.
- Yoga invites you to sharpen your awareness of the present moment, both mentally and physically.
- Yoga is low-impact, which protects the joints from excessive jarring, especially in those with osteoarthritis.
- Yoga improves balance skills, which helps to prevent falls.
- Yoga provides a wide variety of stimulation and demand on the body as compared to repetitive sports or workout machines. Demand makes the bones grow stronger.

- Yoga practice calms the mind, reducing stress.
- Yoga can be practiced alone or in a group. When you practice at home, you can choose your time of day and duration. When you take a class, you receive social support from the group and, ideally, direct instruction from your teacher.
- Yoga, like other forms of exercise, promotes independence and well-being.

Be sure to consult your physician for guidance regarding diet and other lifestyle factors that are involved with bone health and balance.

Fall Prevention Is Fracture Prevention

It's wise to do all we can to avoid fractures. Since most fractures occur from falling, a well-designed yoga practice should address fall prevention in any aspect of your life—moving around your home, walking outside, doing exercise, etc. We need to include all the elements of balancing in our practice: strength, flexibility and coordination. To catch ourselves when we fall, we need flexibility and coordination to regain our balance. If we do fall, we need upper body strength to catch ourselves. And the bonus is, when we develop these skills, we contribute to our agility in daily life.

Remember that your DEXA score is not the only factor to consider in assessing the risk of injuring yourself by falling. Other factors include:

- **Your age.** The risk of fracture increases with each decade.
- **Your hormones.** Hormonal changes contribute to bone loss for both genders.
- **Your eyesight and hearing.** These senses are a big part of regulating balance.
- **Your body awareness.** We need to know where we are in space to keep our balance.
- **Your activity level.** Being active develops bone and muscle strength, body awareness, and nervous system stimulation.

- **Your bone quality.** A bone's inner structure is an indicator of its ability to sustain a fall without fracturing.
- **Your posture.** A chronically stooped posture will predispose you to falls.
- **Your lifestyle factors.** Your job, home environment, and nutrition all play a role in your safety.
- **Your strength, stamina and flexibility.** These traits are developed with a well-designed yoga practice.

If you want a quantitative way to evaluate your risk, medical researchers have developed fracture risk calculation tools, which are available online.[8]

Body Awareness

To prevent falls, we need to develop our body awareness, which is especially important for those with osteoporosis and osteopenia. One crucial aspect of body awareness is "proprioception," the sense of where our body parts are in space and how they move. A healthy nervous system constantly sends input to the brain from receptors in our muscles, tendons and joints. Unfortunately, the aging process can decrease the efficiency of this communication, causing a gradual loss of awareness and control of our posture, balance and movements.

Another aspect of body awareness is "interoception." This is the awareness of processes going on in our internal world, such as our heart rate, breathing or other physical sensations.

Proprioception and interoception decline with age, but only if you let them. The good news is that we can slow the decline of both through physical activity, especially one that encourages moment to moment awareness. Yoga is such an activity; as we practice, we remain alert and aware of what we are doing and how we are doing it. It's not a mindless workout.

---

8   Aasis Unnanuntana, MD, et al. "The Assessment of Fracture Risk," *The Journal of Bone & Joint Surgery*, vol. 92 no. 3 (March 2010): 743-753. doi.org/10.2106/JBJS.I.00919.

Alignment

What is alignment in the context of exercise? It is the process of adjusting the parts of one's body in relation to each other for maximum safety and efficiency in any position or action. Often, this involves recognizing and counteracting habitual movement or postural patterns that bring us out of optimal alignment.

As you practice the poses presented in this book, you'll see instructions to align your body in specific ways. We're not expecting perfection, but there are biomechanical principles that respect the structure of your joints and muscles to protect you from injury. When your joints are out of alignment, your soft tissue (muscles, tendons, ligaments, fascia) will respond by tightening to counteract the misalignment. This tightness can create lifelong chronic pain and movement restriction. For freedom from pain and efficiency of movement and to improve and maintain your balance, alignment is crucial. And when we are well aligned, our subtle inner energy (or "prana") flows most powerfully.

In broad terms, we consider the placement of the feet, knees, pelvis, spine, shoulders and head. Knowing that we're not looking for perfection, we establish our personal best for daily life and for yoga poses. While it's helpful to have a qualified teacher to give you in-person feedback, the instructions in this book will get you started.

Alignment can change over your lifetime and in different circumstances. In your twenties, it might be easy to have good posture, but as you age, you lose muscular strength and standing tall becomes more of a challenge. Perhaps your spine is more curved and not elongated to its fullest extent. Or perhaps an activity you do frequently predisposes you to a risky alignment that could lead to injuries or falls.

The poses I selected for this book are designed to help you establish an understanding of how to best align your body and strengthen the muscles you need to maintain it. Then you can apply this knowledge to your daily life.

There are many facets to alignment, which we're going to cover in the topics that follow. These include the overall shape of your spine, how your pelvis is positioned, and your core strength. But before we get into the specifics of your body's structure, let's look at two broader aspects of yoga technique: form and action, and stability and mobility.

Form and Action

The "form" of a pose is its shape, including the position of your legs, torso, head and arms. For example, the form of the cobra pose has your legs and pelvis flat on the floor, facing downward, while your torso and head lift up with the help of your arms. There is a lot more to know about the details of each form, but for now, it's enough to say that we recognize each pose as distinct from the others by its form.

What I call "action" is the energy and work we add into the shape. With actions, the pose comes to life and your understanding of your body expands. Without actions, it's just the positioning of your body in space.

You'll see instructions, like "Spread your toes" or "Lift your spine up and out of your pelvis" or "Squeeze your shoulder blades toward your spine." These are actions that take us beyond our habits, making the poses safer, transformational and more enjoyable. And it gives us a variety of things to work with, keeping us in the present moment and fully involved in what we're doing.

Often these instructions are expressed in pairs of opposites, such as "Contract your arm muscles to pull your arms into the shoulder joints, then expand out through your fingertips." (See "Stability and Mobility" on page 10.) You might ask, "How can I do these two opposite actions at once?" I encourage you to try it and see for yourself that it is possible and to feel how it enlivens the pose.

This leads us to the second aspect of the practice, which involves our intention.

Stability and Mobility

Are you practicing yoga to be stronger or to be more flexible? Hopefully, the answer to that question is "Both!" (You don't have to choose one or the other.)

In every pose, we create stability first with good alignment and muscular strength to avoid risking injury from overstretching or falling out of a pose. Then, with that as our foundation, we can work on flexibility and mobility, ideally little by little.

Spinal Curves

As we address the topic of alignment, some anatomy review is helpful. The spine is the framework that supports your entire body. Any misalignment of the vertebrae can cause significant problems that hinder your range of motion and other body functions. Therefore, it's important that the vertebrae are properly aligned.

When viewed from the side, the spine is designed to have natural curves. These curvatures give the spine springiness, which protects the skull and brain from the impact of walking, running or jumping.

It's worthwhile to identify these four curves by name, since one of them, kyphosis, is particularly relevant to osteoporosis.

Starting from the top and observing from the side, the first seven vertebrae in the neck (known as the "cervical spine") are rounded toward the front of the body. This is called "lordosis."

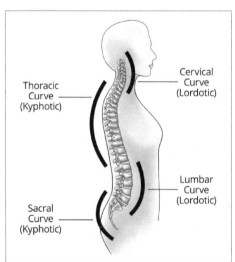

The twelve vertebrae between your waist and your neck (called the "thoracic spine") have a curve known as "kyphosis." This curvature is rounded toward the back of the body, making space for your heart and lungs.

The five vertebrae of your lower back (the "lumbar spine") have a lordotic curve, balancing the same type of shape in your neck.

The lowest five vertebrae at the base of the spine (the "sacral spine") are fused together and are known as the sacrum. Below that is the tailbone (or "coccyx") comprised of several more smaller vertebrae. These form a kyphotic curve like the thoracic spine.

You might wonder, how much curvature should I have in each of these areas? There is not an absolute answer to that question. The same terms, "lordosis" and "kyphosis," are used to identify a normal amount of curve and also an excessive amount. Each of us has a characteristic curvature, and there is quite a bit of variation within what's considered normal.

However, as we age, gravity takes its toll, and arguably the most common deviation of spinal curvature is increased thoracic kyphosis. It's often called "hyperkyphosis" (or more commonly, "dowager's hump"), an extreme rounded shape in the upper back. It is often accompanied by a flattening of the lordotic curve of the lower back. If you have chronic back pain, you might consult a health practitioner or yoga therapist to help you understand how your spinal curves might be contributing to your pain.

The problem with hyperkyphosis is that it creates increased pressure on the front of the vertebrae, which could lead to a wedge fracture (see page 20). If you have osteoporosis and hyperkyphosis in your upper back, some intervention is necessary. The solution yoga offers is to strengthen the upper back with safe back-bending poses, and with that strength, to bring more length to the whole spine, reducing kyphosis and the likelihood of a wedge fracture. It's not easy at first, but your posture and breathing will noticeably improve.

The curves we've looked at so far are related to when the spine is viewed from the side, but there may also be curves when it's viewed from the back. This sideways curvature is called "scoliosis." The locations and degree of the curves differ from one person to another. Mild curvature is very common, and it will not prevent you from exercising or practicing yoga. It is best to consult an experienced teacher in person to evaluate your spine for this condition and give you detailed guidance about your practice. But you can confidently practice the poses in this book because many of them focus on elongating the spine, which is beneficial for those with scoliosis.[9]

With a well-planned and carefully performed yoga regimen, we work to encourage movement in every part of the spine. It's common to move primarily in the areas that activate easily, which are usually the neck and lower back. But we can gradually learn to involve all parts of the spine with yoga.

---

9   If you want more information, I recommend reading *Yoga for Scoliosis* by Elise Browning Miller and nancy DL heraty (nancy heraty, 2016) or *Yoga and Scoliosis* by Marcia Monroe (DemosHealth, 2012).

Pelvic Tilt

In yoga, as in any exercise modality, it's important to notice the position of your pelvis in your body alignment. This determines your spinal curves, since the pelvis is literally the foundation of the spine.

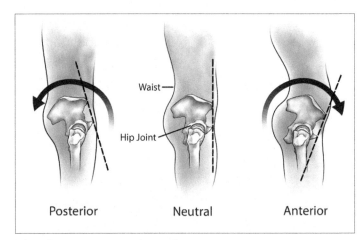

Some of us have a significant lordosis in the lumbar spine. This means, when looking from the side, the top of the pelvis is in front of the bottom of the pelvis, which is called an "anterior tilt." Too much of this can lead to compression of the vertebrae of the lower back and possibly back pain.

Others have the reverse: the tailbone and hip joints thrust forward, the top of the pelvis moves back, and the lower back is flattened. Too much of this tilt puts strain on the mid-back, compresses the sacroiliac joint, and tightens the front of the hip joints. This is called "posterior tilt."

Generally, the anterior tilt is more common in younger people, and the posterior tilt in older people. The ideal alignment is a position in the middle of these two extremes—again, we are trying to find a place in the middle of two opposites. This is called a "neutral pelvis." I'll describe how to find the neutral pelvis in detail later in "Neutral Pelvis" on page 46. It is relevant—even essential—in nearly every pose in this book.

Core Strength

The prevailing definition of "core" according to Merriam-Webster is "the muscles of the mid-region of the torso," which many interpret to mean the abdominal muscles. I believe that, within the fitness and medical communities, there is a tendency to overemphasize abdominal strengthening through sit-ups, crunches or some variation of these common exercises. For anyone with low bone density, this type of exercise is dangerous because it puts excess pressure on the front of the vertebrae as you round your spine quickly and forcefully.

But there is a more comprehensive way to understand the core. It's actually all the muscle groups that make up the middle part of the body, including those of the spine, hips, pelvic floor, thighs and abdominal wall. These core muscles stabilize our body on all sides, creating a source and center for the movements of the rest of the body. This view of the core also prevents a dangerous, but common, tendency to overuse the abdominal muscles when working to strengthen the core.

Stabilizing your core is a fluid and dynamic process, responding to what you are doing at each moment. With a weak core, your body will find other, less efficient strategies for stability, such as tensing your shoulders. With a strong core, you'll be safer in any situation, especially vigorous activities—but also for daily chores or extensive sitting at work. And most of all, you'll have better balance.

One action that may be unfamiliar to most people starting yoga is to lift the pelvic floor. This involves a muscular network at the base of your pelvis that we use to stabilize our center in the yoga poses. Right now, as you're reading, squeeze your pelvic floor and see how it feels. Notice that you can continue to breathe while firming those muscles. You can squeeze toward the center, and then gently lift that floor upward. Try this for fifteen seconds at a time at first, and then gradually integrate it into your practice. As an additional benefit, having a strong pelvic floor may help prevent incontinence.

Tips for Improving Alignment

Remember, to improve and maintain your balance, which is what we'll focus on next, alignment is crucial. So here's a list summarizing the essential reminders, from the foundation provided by your feet to the crown of your head. You'll see these mentioned again in the instructions for each pose as well.

Be patient with yourself as you gradually learn these alignments and apply them appropriately. Mastering them requires a balance of awareness, conscious choice and effort.

- Balance your weight evenly on your feet, aligning the midline of each foot parallel to the other. If your habit is to turn your feet inward or outward, gradually work to become more familiar with this neutral position.

- Direct your knees toward your second and third toes, whether your legs are bent or straight.
- Adjust the tilt of your pelvis until it is appropriate for your body and the pose you are doing.
- Create a slight arch in your lower back and engage your abdominal muscles to support it.
- When doing any forward-bending pose, fold forward from the hips, keeping your spine long and strong without rounding it. This is hip flexion without spinal flexion.
- Lift and broaden your chest, squeezing your shoulder blades together to support your upper back.
- Align your head over your spine as much as possible. If you tend to carry your head forward, pull it back so your head is over your spine, then lift your chin to recover the slight arch in your neck.
- Lengthen your spine and maintain an upright posture while twisting.
- When doing back-bending poses, ensure all parts of the spine are participating, not just those that move easily.

Invigorate your whole body with the energy from your breathing and your highest intention for your well-being.

Balance

As we age, our perceptual and cognitive functions may decline. What that means is our vision and our ability to make quick decisions may be less reliable. But evidence shows that these conditions can be at least partially reversed by regular exercise. The brain can keep learning!

To help us maintain balance, we have three mechanisms in the body that work simultaneously, moment to moment.

First, our **proprioception** sends neural signals from our muscles and joints to the brain that indicate what position we are in. For this to work well, we need sufficient focus to receive those signals and make adjustments when needed. Unfortunately, many older adults have reduced proprioception and possibly also peripheral neuropathy, which is a lack of sensation and motor control in the extremities. Our feet may feel numb or be unable to move easily.

Second, the delicate structures in the **inner ear** respond to changes of position (particularly of the head) and communicate with the brain. This is called the "vestibular system," and it deteriorates with the aging process, causing hearing loss and a decline in spatial orientation and postural control.

Third, our **vision** gives us a sense of orientation to the surrounding environment. We need to remember to sharpen our attention and our visual focus (both direct and peripheral), whether walking on the street, moving around house, or doing any kind of exercise. This may seem obvious, but ask yourself: how often do I get lost in my thoughts while doing my daily activities? If that inattention becomes a persistent habit, it can increase your risk of falling.

If you suddenly develop a balance issue, such as dizziness or light-headedness when transitioning from lying down to standing up, or if you have reduced sensation in your feet, I recommend you seek medical help to test for inner ear, neuropathy or cardiovascular issues. Many common medications may also affect balance skills. However, a gradual development of balance problems is most likely to be caused by our normal aging process. This is where yoga can help.

With yoga, you improve your proprioception, strengthen your muscles, and increase your flexibility. I've mentioned why proprioception and muscle strength are important. But why flexibility? When you sense that your balance is off, the natural tendency is to adjust your position to regain your balance. This could be catching yourself with one foot after tripping over an obstacle or widening your stance while walking down the aisle of a fast-moving train. To do that, you need fast responses, but also hip and leg mobility. Flexibility allows you a greater range of adaptive moves to steady yourself and prevent a fall. For this reason, I've included an exercise for dynamic balancing (on page 68), which I believe is just as important as learning to balance on one foot in stillness.

Tips for Developing Better Balance

If you want to develop better balance, here are a few things to remember.

- At first, wear good shoes for your practice if your balance is significantly challenged. Then progress to practicing with bare feet.

- Be aware of your feet and use the four corners exercise (page 50) to align them.

- Use an appropriate support, like a wall or the back of a chair. Gradually increase the challenge by decreasing your dependence on it.

- Develop a strong core, which includes your spinal muscles, hips, thighs, abdominals and pelvic floor.

- Use your visual focus—first keeping it straight ahead, then challenging yourself by looking in different directions while in a pose.

For further information on studies of balance, check out these sources:

Sloan, Erica. "Here's Why Maintaining Your Balancing Skills as You Age Is Tied to Longevity," Well + Good (July 9, 2022). ellensaltonstall.com/longevity.

Gil Araujo, Claudio, et al., "Successful 10-second one-legged stance performance predicts survival in middle-aged and older individuals," British Journal of Sports Medicine, v. 56, no. 17 (June 21, 2022): 975-980. doi.org/10.1136/bjsports-2021-105360.

Chapter 4. Before You Begin

While you may be tempted to get started with your new yoga practice right away, it's important to discuss any restrictions you may have with members of your healthcare team first. This includes physicians, physical therapists, and experienced yoga and movement teachers.

If you have any injuries or chronic conditions, know your limitations and adapt for them. Take special care if you have spinal disc problems, blood pressure issues, or a recent surgery or illness.

I have shared a few specific cautions for those with osteoporosis or osteopenia below. However, considering every possible condition, injury or disease is beyond the scope of this book. Use your common sense and consult with your medical practitioner. We'll also establish some guidelines for your practice and discuss props you may want to use to help maximize the benefit of the poses.

Cautions for Those with Low Bone Density

If you have osteoporosis or osteopenia:

- **Avoid spinal flexion** (bending forward), especially with force. Two notable examples of this are moving quickly to reach for your toes and doing sit-ups.
- **Avoid risky balancing.** Practice with the support of a wall or the back of a chair at first, then gradually increase the challenge by touching the support with only one finger.

- **When twisting, make sure your spine is long and tall.** Spinal twists are beneficial, but only if done correctly. Use your back and abdominal muscles to perform the movement instead of forcing a deeper twist with your arms.
- **When practicing forward-bending poses,** take special care to begin with an anterior tilt of your pelvis (shifting your weight to the front of your sitting bones) and lengthen your spine upward. Prepare by stretching your hamstring muscles (at the back of your thighs) while lying on your back. (For example, by doing leg stretches with a belt, as shown on page 78.) While this is an exercise I always recommend, this stretch is especially important for those with low bone density.
- **When practicing back-bending poses,** spread the effort throughout the spine, not just where it's easy to move.

Guidelines for Your Practice

When you're ready to start, consider the following guidelines to get the most out of your yoga experience.

- **Time your normal cycles of breathing** to determine how many breaths you take in fifteen to thirty seconds. This is the minimum time to hold each pose, if possible, for maximum benefit. By keeping track of how many breaths you take within this time frame and counting them during a pose, you can effectively time yourself without relying on a watch or clock.
- **Always use your breath** to focus, energize and release. Staying in touch with your breathing is an essential part of yoga practice. When you are distracted, bring your awareness back to your breath to recover your focus. If your energy lags, breathe in more vigorously and feel how it enlivens you. When you confront discomfort from tight muscles and joints, exhale more fully to prompt your nervous system to release mentally and physically. For more information on breathing, refer to my article "Breath is Food for the Body and Soul" (ellensaltonstall. com/breath).

- **Be curious.** Remember what my teacher Mary Dunn said: "First you get to know the poses, then you get to know yourself in the poses."
- **Honestly consider** your level of strength and coordination as you design your practice. If you're a beginner, for the first few weeks, practice the poses in Chapters 5 through 10 and end with a cool-down pose from Chapter 12. This will create a strong foundation. Then add the standing poses from Chapter 11 a few at a time. If you are an experienced practitioner, consider how to get the satisfaction of the practice you love without the risks. The goal is to avoid injury while challenging yourself gradually.
- **For a daily practice,** I suggest you warm-up with at least two of the sequences (from Chapters 6 through 8). Then choose four or five of the standing poses, altering your choices each time you practice. Be sure to include at least one balancing pose in your daily regimen as well. To end your practice, choose one or two cool-down poses.
- **In all poses,** prioritize muscular strength and precise alignment over flexibility. Remember, *how* you do the poses is every bit as important as *which* poses you do.

Whenever a pose offers multiple variations, they are listed in order starting with the least challenging and building from there. The first variation often uses props that provide support and comfort as you grow accustomed to the pose and increase your strength. These variations often help you to learn the body positions without requiring too much in terms of balance, strength or flexibility. But as you develop those traits, subsequent variations help you to continue to grow your stamina and abilities. When props are used in a later variation, it's often to deepen the stretching involved in the pose.

Props

We use props in yoga to assist in creating the optimal alignment while working at our level. Depending on your body proportions and flexibility, you might always choose to use a prop for some poses. While some people may think of using props as a "cop-out," they actually help you work more fully and accurately. One of my teachers called props "our silent teachers." We learn from the support they give us. Each posture reveals several challenges, such as tight hips, a weak spine, or poor balance. With the right prop, you reduce one challenge in order to focus on another.

For instance, if you're doing a standing pose that requires one or both hands to come to the floor, tight hamstrings can be a significant obstacle. Resting your hands on blocks, or even a chair, will help tremendously. Or if you're doing a seated pose and your pelvis can't tilt anteriorly enough to support a lifted spine, sitting on a folded blanket can help you achieve that lift. When you are learning a balance pose, touching a wall or a chair helps you to remain steady for a longer time.

Use discernment to determine the most important actions in any pose and consider how a prop might help you. Note any discomforts and limitations, and see if a prop gives you more confidence, even when you're challenged. With the help of these aids, you can progress intelligently in your practice.

The most common prop associated with yoga is a yoga mat, which provides both cushioning and a nonslip surface when your feet or hands are your foundation.

However, there are other props I recommend having for your practice too. Here's a short list of them and how to use them.

- **Two blocks** to provide a lift to support your hands, your pelvis or your head when reaching the floor is challenging or creates a misalignment.
- **A chair** to perform some seated and several standing poses. Ideally, it should be without arms, such as a sturdy folding chair.
- **A long belt** for two important practices: the shoulder halter, which aligns your shoulders and upper back, and the supine leg stretches, which improve your hip mobility.
- **Blankets, bolsters and towels** to create padding for various poses and relaxing comfort in the cool-down poses.
- **A wall** to provide support and stability in some poses.

> If you're looking for a good place to buy yoga equipment, I recommend yogaaccessories.com and huggermugger.com.

If you don't have the recommended props, here are some suitable substitutes.

- To substitute for a yoga mat, you can do standing poses with shoes on.
- To substitute for blocks, use a stack of books.
- To substitute for a long belt, you can use a bathrobe belt.
- To substitute for a blanket, bolster or towels, you can use pillows.
- To substitute for a wall, you can use a sturdy bookshelf, countertop or chair back.

Bodymind Ballwork

In addition to yoga, I teach a bodywork technique I developed called "Bodymind Ballwork." In this technique, we use rubber balls of varying textures and sizes (from as small as a walnut to as big as a melon) to highlight, support, massage and stretch localized areas of the body. The balls directly address tight connective tissues and muscles, restoring healthy circulation and seamless movement between their layers.

I have identified specific balls I feel are best to use, and there are many options that suit different body types, goals and varieties of pressure. They're not one size fits all. Alternatively, you can practice with tennis balls.

There are techniques for every part of the body, from your head to your toes. The result is a wonderful feeling of spaciousness, lightness and ease in the body and a quiet alertness in the mind.

> If you're looking for a good place to buy rubber balls to use in Bodymind Ballwork, I recommend lifesaball.org.

You can significantly improve your balance by working on the bottoms of your feet with a small ball about the size of a walnut. This wakes up your proprioception and subtle movement potential, making it possible for you to use your feet effectively for balance.

The name "Bodymind Ballwork" is used to underscore the truth that all experiences register in the body and the mind simultaneously. Working on the body will shift our mental state, and mental focus will shift our physical state. As humans, we are already mentally and physically integrated—meaning that

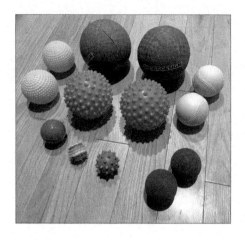

the mind and body are intricately connected from one moment to the next. But we don't always feel that way.

This technique is an elegantly simple and profound pathway to the experience of an integrated self. When combined with yoga, you will have a way to loosen areas of the body that are stiff, making the practice more enjoyable and beneficial.

If you're interested in exploring Bodymind Ballwork, you can find out more on my website at ellensalton-stall.com/ballwork, my YouTube channel (ellensalton-stall.com/youtube), or in my book, *The Bodymind Ballwork Method*.

Lexicon

Asana is a Sanskrit word that translates as "seat" and denotes a body position, pose or posture. It is pronounced "AH-suh-nuh" and is the suffix at the end of the Sanskrit names of yoga poses.

Arch is commonly used to describe extension of the spine, lengthening in the front (for example, when arching your back to look upward).

Curve has two meanings in the context of the human body. First, it is a general term referring to a shape that deviates from a straight line. In the case of the spine, it is commonly used to describe the natural shapes of the spine. (See the figure on page 25.) Second, it is commonly used as a synonym for flexion of the spine, such as bending forward and rounding the spine to look downward.

Extension has two slightly different meanings as well. First, it is a general term meaning "the act of stretching out to the fullest length." Second, it is a particular joint movement that increases the angle in the front of the body between two or more bones. It also can denote a return from flexion back to a neutral position of the joint. For example, when we stand after sitting in a chair, we are extending our hip joints, bringing them back to neutral after flexing them to sit down. When we kick a ball, we first flex the knee, then extend it forcefully.

Flexion is the bending of a joint that decreases the angle between the bones of the joint. For example, when you sit, that's hip flexion. When you bring one arm forward to give someone a handshake, that's shoulder flexion. Spinal flexion is a forward-moving curve of the vertebral spine, which has twenty-four small segments. When many of these joints go into flexion, the result is a rounded shape, rather than the angular shape of hip flexion.

Hip flexion, see flexion.

Isometric translates as "same length." When we work isometrically in the poses, we contract our muscles but no movement occurs at the joints involved. We use this in yoga frequently to hold the poses. For instance, we use the front thigh muscles isometrically to hold our knees bent at a certain angle, opposing the force of gravity that would pull us down and bend the knees farther. In the outer thigh strengthening exercise (page 52), we use our hip muscles to counter the opposite push from our hands and only a slight movement occurs in the hips.

Midline divides the body into right and left halves.

Pelvic tilt is the spatial position of the pelvis in relation to the lower back and the thighs.

Pronation is the position of your forearm and hand when the palm is turned downward.

Prone is the position of lying down with the front of your body facing the floor.

Spinal flexion, see flexion.

Supination is the position of your forearm and hand when the palm is turned upward.

Supine is the position of lying down with the front of your body facing upward.

Suggested Sequences

The time required to practice each of these sequences will vary from one person to the next, based on your experience level with the material. Use your discretion to adapt the sequence to fill the time you have. I recommend building up your practice to thirty to forty-five minutes a day.

When you are just getting started, the first few items on each week's list may be all you can manage or have time for. As you progress, you'll be able to add more poses and expand the time.

Week 1

1. All fundamentals
2. All standing warm-ups
3. All supine series
4. Selected prone series
   - Cat/cow
   - Plank pose
   - Downward-facing dog
   - Cobra pose
   - Child's pose

Week 2

1. All standing warm-ups
2. All supine series
3. Selected prone series
   - Cat/cow
   - Downward-facing dog
   - Cobra pose
   - Low lunge with backbend
   - Child's pose
4. All chair series
5. Selected standing poses
   - Mountain pose
   - Chair pose
   - Leaning goddess pose
   - Warrior 2
6. One cool-down pose
   - Corpse pose with legs on chair

Week 3

1. Review fundamentals
2. All supine series
3. Selected prone series
   - Balancing table pose
   - Downward-facing dog
   - Locust pose
   - Child's pose
4. All wrist and hand series
5. Selected standing series
   - Leaning goddess
   - Warrior 2
   - Side angle pose
   - Wide-legged standing forward bend
6. One cool-down pose
   - Mountain brook pose

Week 4

1. All standing warm-ups
2. All supine series
3. Selected prone series
   - Downward-facing dog
   - Plank pose
   - Locust pose
   - Child's pose
4. All wrist and hand series
5. Selected standing series
   - Mountain pose
   - Leaning goddess
   - Tree pose
   - Triangle pose
   - Half moon pose
   - Wide-legged standing forward bend
6. One cool-down pose
   - Corpse pose with legs on chair

Week 5

1. All supine series
2. Selected prone series
   - Downward-facing dog
   - Low lunge with backbend
   - Child's pose
3. All chair series
4. Selected standing series
   - Mountain pose
   - One-legged standing twist
   - Warrior 1
   - Warrior 3
   - Wide-legged standing forward bend
5. One cool-down pose
   - Corpse pose with legs on chair

Week 6

1. All supine series
2. All prone series
3. Selected standing series
   - Chair pose
   - Tree pose
   - Triangle pose
   - Half moon pose
   - Revolved triangle pose
   - Revolved side angle pose
   - Wide-legged standing forward bend
4. Two cool-down poses
   - Child's pose
   - Mountain brook

After that, make your own sequences!

Chapter 5. Fundamentals

Learning the fundamentals of yoga is essential because it lays the foundation for a safe and fulfilling practice. Understanding the basics will help prevent injuries and ensures you reap the full benefits of each pose. These essentials provide the skills that set the stage for growth, confidence and a transformative yoga experience.

Neutral Pelvis

Knowing how to find a neutral position for your pelvic tilt is essential to nearly every yoga pose you may ever do since it's the foundation for stability. People often sit and stand with a predominantly posterior tilt, which rounds the spine, creating a slumped posture. This exercise shows you the two opposite movements, anterior and posterior (or front and back), and how to find a neutral place in the middle.

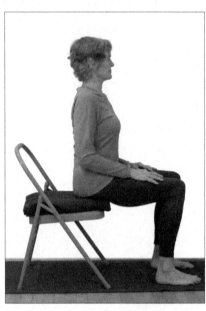

Benefit: To feel how the pelvis and lower spine work together to build strength and coordinated balance

Props: A chair

Finer Points

- When you find your neutral pelvic tilt while sitting, notice how the contact with the chair helps you to feel the sitting bones clearly.
- When you do this action while standing, keep your legs as steady as possible as you move your pelvis.

Instructions

1. Sitting at the front edge of the chair, feel your sitting bones against the seat.
2. Shift your weight from side to side.
3. While one side is lifted, use your hand to pull that buttock to the back and side.
4. Repeat the movement with the other buttock.

   Notice that this adjustment makes the top of your pelvis tip forward and your pubic bone downward, causing your lower back to arch into an anterior tilt. This tilt will help you elongate your spine.
5. Roll backward on your sitting bones into the posterior tilt and notice how that affects your spine. Does it round backward? Does your torso become shorter?

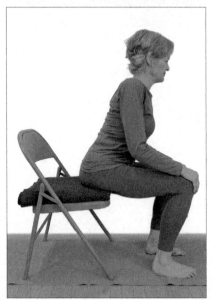

From this experimentation, you can feel how those two opposing tilts determine the alignment of the pelvis and lower back.

6. Lean forward and feel the difference between the anterior and posterior tilt in this position.

7. Stand and do those same two movements, noticing how the pelvic tilt changes your posture.

Feel how the anterior tilt moves your upper pelvis forward and your thighs back and how the posterior tilt flattens the lower back and pushes your thighs forward.

Observe which one of these tilts seems habitual to you. Is one easier than the other? This is your natural tilt, which may not be optimal for your overall alignment.

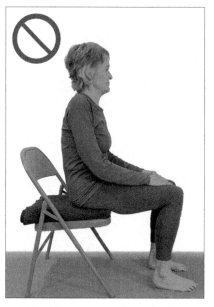

8. Find your neutral tilt, which is a balance of the anterior and posterior tilts. Experiment with using different amounts of lower abdominal support to find what works best for you. There's no exact position to hold; rather, it's a dynamic process.

Reflections

- What is your habitual posture in your pelvis and lower back when you are sitting and standing?
- What do you notice about the relationship between your pelvic tilt and your spine?
- Can you bend forward from your hips without curving your spine?
- Do you feel the tilts differently on your left and right sides of the pelvis? (This is normal.)

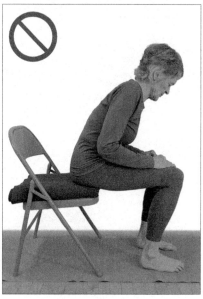

Abdominal and Pelvic Floor Strength

Abdominal and pelvic floor strength is key to protecting and strengthening your lower back, especially when it's done without spinal flexion.

Benefit: To become adept at using strong abdominal support without flexing the spine

Props: A yoga mat

Finer Points

- Notice how a strong core supports the natural curve of your lower spine.

Instructions

1. Lie on your mat on your back with knees bent.
2. Do a few pelvic tilting movements, ending with a neutral pelvis and your lower back slightly off the floor.
3. Carefully contract your abdominal muscles and pelvic floor without changing your pelvic tilt or flexing your spine. In other words, don't let your waist press onto the mat. You might want to put a towel under it the first few times you try this.

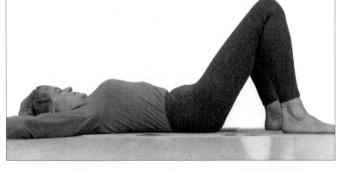

4. Stand and practice this some more. Find the neutral pelvic tilt and contract your abdominals and pelvic floor without flexing your spine.

Reflections

- Can you continue your normal breathing rhythm as you do this exercise?
- How does your awareness of this strength show up in your daily movements?

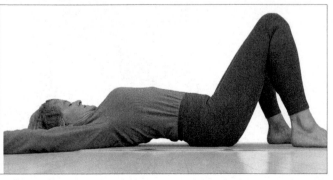

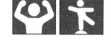

The Shoulder Halter

The shoulder halter gives the experience of healthy shoulder and neck alignment, promoting a sense of stability and mobility in your upper body.

Benefit: To improve upper back, shoulder and neck alignment

Props: A long yoga belt (8–10′)

Finer Points

- Imagine how this posture can affect your daily life!

Instructions

1. Standing tall, bring the middle of the belt behind your upper back, wrap the ends under your armpits, and bring them forward, one on each side.
2. Keeping some tension on the belt, carefully bring each side back over the shoulder it's currently in the front of.
3. Cross the belt behind your neck and let the ends hang down near the sides of your hips.
4. Grasp one tail with each hand near your hips.
5. Inhale and expand your upper torso with your breath while pulling down on the tails of the belt at the same time. Remain like this for several moments.
6. Walk around to feel this alignment in movement.
7. When you remove the belt, see how much of this alignment you can retain in your upper back, shoulders and neck.

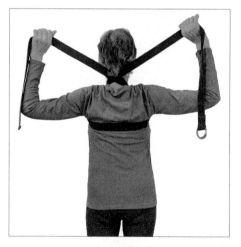

Reflections

- Are your shoulders farther back than usual?
- Is your neck longer?
- Is your upper back more lifted?
- Does this feel different from your usual posture?

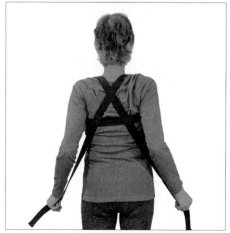

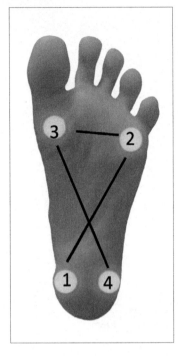

The Four Corners of the Feet

The four corners of your feet include the base of the big and pinky toes, as well as the inner and outer parts of the heel. When you press gently through these, it helps create a stable foundation for your posture and poses.

Benefit: To balance your weight well and strengthen your foot muscles.

Props: A yoga mat (optional)

Finer Points

- When working with one foot, avoid the common tendency for the rest of your body to tense up as you concentrate.

Instructions

1. Begin by standing normally and feel the balance of your weight on your two feet. Do you tend to place more weight on one foot or the other? Or on one part of the foot?

2. Working with one foot at a time, stand with most of your weight on that foot.

3. With the other, tilt your foot so the inner heel is the only part touching the floor.

4. Keeping that part down, touch the base of your little toe (the joint at its base) to the floor. Notice how various muscles in the sole of your foot (called "intrinsic muscles") are working as you do these steps. Don't worry if this is hard to do. Treat it as a fun challenge!

5. Keeping those two points down, stretch across the ball of your foot to bring the base of your big toe to the floor. Notice how it feels to widen your foot in this way.

6. With those three points staying in place, press your outer heel down.
   Feel how your weight balances on these four corners. As you stand on one foot, experiment by moving through the sequence like an internal dance.

7. Repeat this sequence with your other foot.

8. When you stop doing this as an exercise, notice how your weight balances on your feet.

Reflections

- How do your feet feel differently after doing this?
- Which corners are easiest for you to find and press down? Which are less easy?
- What does this tell you about your usual posture on your feet?
- What do you feel in your knees and hips as you do this exercise?

Knee Tracking

It's important to pay attention to knee alignment to avoid injury and protect the structures of the joint. For proper positioning, your knee should always track toward your second or third toe.

Benefit: To align your knees well as they bend, for safety and strength

Props: A yoga mat (optional)

Finer Points

- Spread your toes for better awareness.

Instructions

1. Stand with your feet balanced on their four corners and place them hip-width apart.
2. Bend your knees and look to see where your kneecaps are pointing.
3. Adjust them as needed so they point toward the second or third toe.
4. Practice this several times, observing the knees as they bend.

Reflections

- Do you find your knees tend to turn toward each other when you bend them?
- What do you have to do differently to align your knees to point them toward your second or third toes?
- Where do you feel the actions needed to align your knees to face straight ahead?

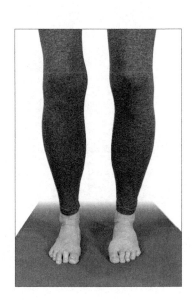

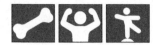

Outer Thigh Strengthening

As you get older, the muscle strength in your outer thighs may decline, which can make everyday activities harder. Lateral movements hone your outer quads, the sides of your hips, and your glutes. Strengthening these muscles can counteract age-related weakness, prevent loss of independence, and improve alignment and balance.

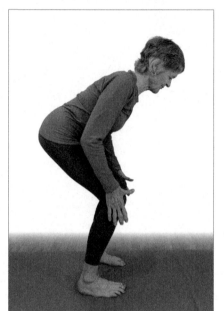

Benefit: To strengthen the outer hip muscles for good lower body support and balance

Props: A belt (optional)

Finer Points

- Notice the contraction of the muscles in your outer hips. These are the abductor muscles, which widen the thighs and the sitting bones by pulling them away from the midline. They are very important for balance.

Instructions

1. Stand with your feet hip-width apart.
2. Bend at your hips and knees, placing your hands on the outsides of your knees.
3. Make your spine long and strong, creating flexion at the hips without spinal flexion.
4. With your hands, push your knees toward the midline. At the same time, push outward isometrically with your thighs using equal pressure. Your knees will not move, but your sitting bones will widen.
5. Hold this action for several breaths.
6. When you're done, return to standing.

Standing Variation with a Belt

1. Make a loop with the belt that encircles your legs just below the knees when your feet are hip-width apart. The belt will stabilize your lower legs.

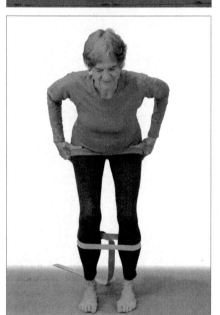

2. With your knees slightly bent, strongly widen your thighs, keeping your weight on the four corners of your feet.

3. Hold the pose for a few breaths.

4. When you're done, return to standing.

Reflections

- Feeling these muscles working is a new experience for many people. What does it feel like to you?

- Can you feel how this will help you align your knees toward the second or third toe?

Stabilizing and Expanding Energies

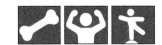

Energy is an important concept in yoga. Stabilizing energy focuses on strength and integration, while expanding energy stretches the body and increases the sense of "flow." Although beginning yoga students will need to practice these two energy states separately, more experienced practitioners strive to achieve both energy states simultaneously.

Benefit: To create strength and flexibility in every pose

Props: None

Finer Points

- As you learn this, appreciate the muscles you have and how they are working.

- Be confident in your ability to strengthen them.

Instructions

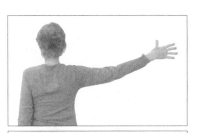

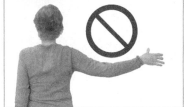

This action can be done with any part of the body, but it's easiest to practice first with your arms. In this way, we engage our full body and mind to achieve a feeling of empowerment.

1. While standing, raise one arm to the side at shoulder height or higher.

2. Contract the muscles around your bones from your fingertips all the way along your arm into your shoulder joint. Create a stabilizing support for the whole arm as you contract the muscles.

Think of plugging your arm into your shoulder joint as you would plug a cord into an outlet. Notice the stabilizing feeling of that action.

3. Keep about 80 percent of the muscular strength you've just activated, but release the tension enough to extend your energy back in the other direction, from your center out through the arm, all the way to your fingertips.

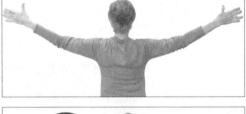

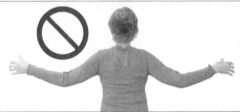

Feel the length and strength of your arm for a few breaths.

4. Lower your arm to your side and feel the energetic awakening.

5. Repeat with your other arm, then try it with both arms at once.

6. When you're ready, release your arms down to your sides.

With those two opposites balanced, you'll have tremendous strength while retaining mobility.

Reflections

- How is this different from making a shape with your body with the least possible effort? How does it feel to you?
- Do you notice a change in your breathing or a particular emotion arising as you do these two opposite actions?

Neck Extension

In many yoga poses, your head will be held off-center. When it's tilting backward, it's important to support the neck with strength from all sides to prevent injury. This exercise gives you a foundational experience of that strength that you can apply to many other poses in this book.

Benefit: To learn how to support the neck for back-bending poses

Props: A yoga mat or chair

Finer Points

- If you have difficulty with your balance, do this exercise while seated.
- Proceed through the steps methodically to experience the greatest benefit.
- Notice how this exercise also affects your shoulders and upper back.

Instructions

1. Place the chair in the middle of the mat with the seat facing a short end.
2. While sitting comfortably in the chair, extend your head and spine up and out of the pelvis. Imagine that the top of your head is floating upward.
3. Squeeze your shoulder blades in toward your spine, which lifts your chest.
4. Touch the top of your neck, where your spine meets your skull.
5. Push your head straight back against your fingers. This will tuck your chin in a bit and engage the front of your neck.
6. Retaining this position, bring your hand back down to your thigh.
7. Lift your chin slightly and look straight ahead.
8. Gradually tilt your head back and extend through its top as if a golden string is pulling your head up and back in a supported arching action. Look up as you do this.
9. Stay with this neck extension for a few breaths, then return to looking straight ahead.

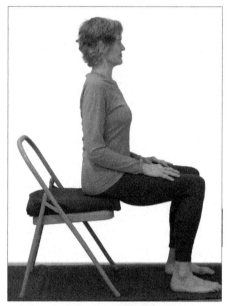

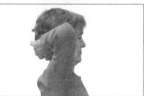

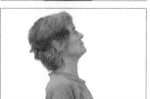

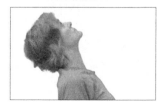

Reflections

- Do you have evenly balanced muscular support on all sides of the neck in this extended position?
- How is this different from the way you might look up in your daily life?

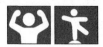

Getting Down on the Floor

Many of the poses in the chapters to come involve getting down on the floor. Since there are many ways to do that, but not all of them are safe, I've provided instructions for how to get into this position without hurting yourself.

Benefit: To safely get onto the floor without spinal flexion or danger of falling

Props: A chair or block

Finer Points

- Keep your spine long through all these steps.
- Use your core muscles to support your lower torso as you change position.
- Practice this movement on both sides to determine which is best for you.
- If you are more flexible, use a block instead of the chair.

Instructions

1. Stand with the chair or block on your right side, about 2–3′ in front of you.
2. Take one long step forward with your left foot, bringing it in line with the chair or block.
3. Bend your left knee and put your right hand on the chair or block, keeping your spine long.
4. Bend your right knee, bringing it down onto the floor or mat.
5. Bring your left knee to the floor next to your right knee and come onto your hands and knees.
6. Lower one hip to the floor by turning your pelvis.
7. Lower your torso to the floor.
8. Roll onto your back and readjust your position on the mat as needed.

Reflections

- How is this different from other ways you have gotten down onto the floor?
- Can you picture being so familiar with doing this that you do it instinctively?

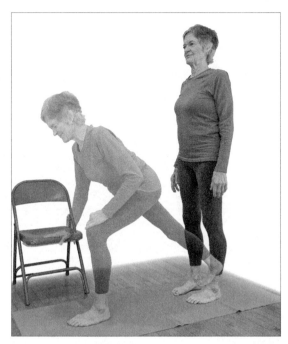

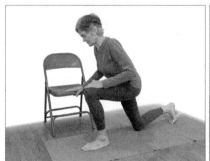
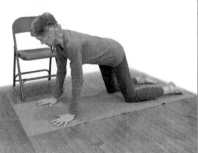
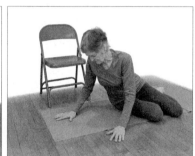

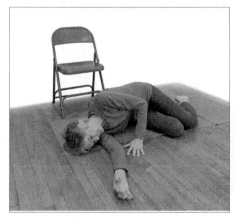
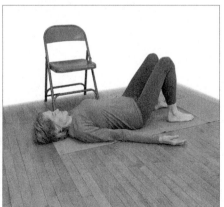

Chapter 6. Standing Warm-Ups

These warm-ups are done while standing to introduce useful concepts about posture for daily life. The included exercises are for strengthening the legs and upper back, along with playful techniques for improving balance. Many of the fundamentals from the previous chapter are brought together in this sequence, leading up to one of the most important poses to practice for bone health: the chair pose.

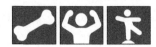

Mountain Pose

Tadasana

tah-DAH-suh-nuh

Mountain pose is often considered the most basic yoga pose, but it can be challenging too. In doing it, we establish the optimum alignment from our feet to the top of our head with care and precision. We can then apply that positioning to all our poses for best results.

Benefit: To practice optimum standing posture for daily life, using all the postural alignments

Props: None

Finer Points

- Be sure to feel your body energized and alive. Make the sum more than the collection of all the parts.

Instructions

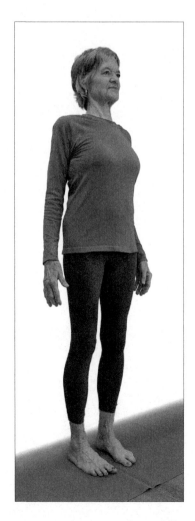

1. Stand with your feet parallel to each other and hip-width apart.
2. Move the tops of your thighs slightly back and notice how your lower back will arch somewhat.
3. Lift your abdomen and lengthen your tailbone without pushing your thighs forward. This is your neutral pelvis.
4. Lift your chest using the strength in your upper back as you lightly squeeze your shoulder blades toward the spine.
5. Let your head float up with ease, lengthening your neck on all sides.
6. Let your arms hang naturally by your hips.
7. Calmly gaze straight ahead and feel the support of your breath. Embody the strength and dignity of a mountain.
8. When you're ready, release the pose.

Reflections

- Can you feel the midline of your body connecting your feet, legs, pelvis, torso and head?
- Do you feel the two flows of energy, stabilizing and expanding, operating in this dignified pose?

Shoulder and Wrist Circles

Our shoulders and wrists are moving all day long, and they are common locations for chronic discomfort and movement restriction. Also, if we find ourselves about to fall, we may reach out to catch ourselves, putting extra demand on the shoulders and wrists. These warm-ups loosen those joints to be ready for more to come.

Benefit: To move with ease in the shoulders and arms

Props: None

Finer Points

- You can do these circles while sitting or standing, whichever you prefer.
- Be sure to isolate the movements where intended and apply a full range of motion at a pace that enables you to feel what's happening.

Instructions

1. Make a slow, careful circle with your shoulders. First bring both sides forward, then up, then back, and release them down. Repeat as many times as you wish.
2. With your arms in a comfortable position, circle your wrists. Again, repeat as many times as you'd like.

Reflections

- Have you noticed any changes in your ease of movement from day to day as you do this exercise?
- Do you find that after these full-range movements, your wrists are less stiff?

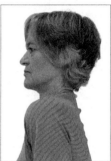
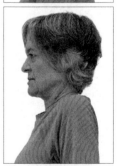
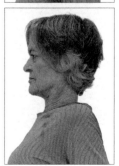

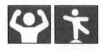

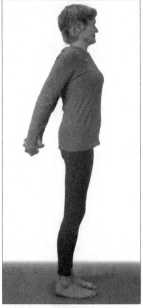

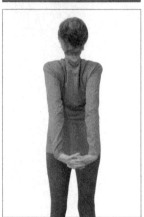

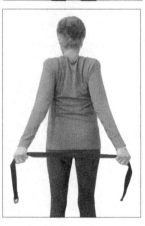

Hands Clasped Behind the Back

Clasping your hands behind your back is one of the easiest exercises to integrate into your normal day. It stretches your shoulders and reminds your upper body to remain open in the front and strong in the back, which helps both your posture and your breathing.

Benefit: To stretch the front of the shoulders and strengthen the upper back, improving posture

Props: None

Finer Points

- To counter the common tendency to push your ribs forward when your shoulders move back, breathe into the back of your ribs.
- If possible, look in a mirror to check both the front and side views. Then you'll be able to see if you can actually move the shoulders back significantly.

Instructions

1. As you stand tall, roll your shoulders back, which will widen your collarbones, bringing them square across the top of your chest.
2. Clasp your hands behind you.
3. With each inhalation, lift and expand your chest, and with each exhalation, squeeze your shoulder blades toward your spine and slightly downward.
4. Hold the pose for a few breaths, looking straight ahead.
5. When you're ready, release the pose.

Variation

As an alternative to clasping your hands, hold onto a belt behind your back.

Reflections

- Where do you feel your muscles working? Where do you feel muscles stretching?
- Do you feel how this exercise uses both the stabilizing and expanding energies?

Pectoral Stretch

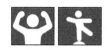

For many of us, our shoulders roll forward from extensive desk work or other tasks. This causes the pectoral muscles in the front of the chest to shorten and remain that way unless challenged in the opposite direction. This stretch counteracts that tendency and gives you more freedom of movement in your shoulders, as well as better posture.

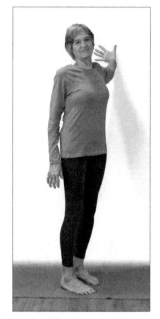

Benefit: To stretch the front shoulder muscles, especially pectoralis major, improving posture

Props: A wall

Finer Points

- Practice the stabilizing and expanding energies in this pose.
- Straighten your arm, but avoid locking your elbow.

Instructions

1. Stand with your left side about 18″ from a wall.
2. Place your left hand on the wall with the fingers pointing either upward or backward. You can have your full hand or only your fingertips touching the wall. It's up to you.
3. Create the balance of stabilizing and expanding energies in your arm for both stability and stretch.
4. Turn your whole body slightly to your right, away from the wall. Stop turning when you feel a good stretch in the shoulder and possibly down the arm.
5. Stay there for several breaths.
6. Release and repeat on the other side.

Reflections

- Can you keep your shoulders away from your ears as you do this?
- Do you feel the stretch differently on your right and left sides?
- Are there specific places in your shoulders or arms that especially feel this stretch?

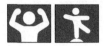

Heel Lift

A heel lift is a simple exercise that refines the action of your ankle muscles for good stability.

Benefit: To strengthen the sides of the ankles for better balance

Props: A wall or the back of a chair and a blanket or pillow (optional)

Finer Points

- Avoid allowing your ankles to shift away from the midline as your heels lift.
- Stabilize your pelvis as you isolate this action in your ankles.

Instructions

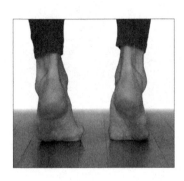

1. Stand facing the wall or next to some other object, such as a table or chair.
2. Touching the support lightly for balance, lift your heels, coming onto the balls of your foot, with your weight concentrated on your first three toes. Feel the supportive action of your ankle muscles on both sides, as you lift the heels straight up.
3. Bring your heels back to the floor and repeat this action several times until your muscles fatigue.

Once you are comfortable with this heel lift, try spreading your toes too.

Variations

- Repeat this technique while standing on one leg at a time. Then switch legs and do it again.
- For a more advanced method, stand on a pillow or folded blanket while doing your heel lifts.

Reflections

- Do you feel this exercise differently on the left and right sides?
- Does this exercise give you more awareness of your ankle alignment and control?

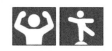

Standing Backbend

Here's another simple exercise you can do anytime during your day to counteract stooped posture and build spinal strength.

Benefit: To strengthen the upper back for postural support

Props: A wall

Finer Points

- If your upper back is difficult to move, keep trying! It will develop little by little.
- Support this expansion with your breath.
- Focus this movement in your middle and upper back, between your waist and your shoulders.

Instructions

There are two variations of this pose: one using a wall and the other without it. The wall gives you a reference that's helpful when you are learning this exercise. Once you've built your confidence, you can do it without the wall.

Variation 1: At the wall

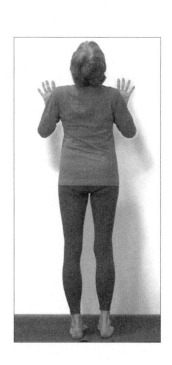

1. Stand facing the wall, about 12″ away from it, and place your hands on it at eye level, shoulder-width apart.
2. Squeeze your shoulder blades together and lift your ribs and collarbones as you inhale.
3. Continue breathing normally.
4. Pull your chin and jaw back to tone the muscles at the front of your neck in preparation for tilting the head backward. (See "Neck Extension" on page 54.)
5. With your hands pressing into the wall and not moving, isometrically pull downward with your hands against the wall. This will lift your ribs up.
6. Tilt your chin to look upward, expanding out through the crown of your head.
7. Simultaneously expand down through your pelvis and legs, and rise up through your upper body.
8. Hold the pose for several breaths, then release when you're ready.

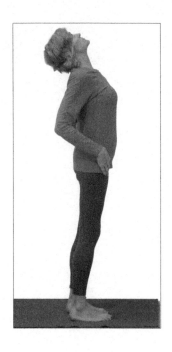

Variation 2: Without the wall

1. Stand tall, establishing the alignments for the mountain pose. (See page 60.)
2. Touch the front of your hips to remind yourself to remain steady there.
3. Lift your spine up and out of the pelvis and contract the muscles along the spine.
4. Squeeze your shoulder blades together as you inhale.
5. Pull your chin and jaw back to tone the muscles at the front of your neck in preparation for tilting the head backward. (See "Neck Extension" on page 54.)
6. With your legs and pelvis steady, lift your chest and tilt your head as if a string is pulling it up and back.
7. Hold the pose for several breaths, then release.

Reflections

- Is there evenly balanced muscular support on all sides of your neck in this extended position?
- Do you feel the stabilizing and expanding energies both working in this pose?

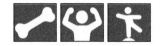

Chair Pose

Utkatasana

oot-kah-TAH-suh-nuh

In the chair pose, you incorporate many of the skills from earlier in this book into one powerful standing pose. Notice how many of the alignments and actions you can do simultaneously.

This is one of the most important poses you can do because it strengthens the bones of your pelvis, spine and legs. It also exemplifies hip flexion without spinal flexion.

The classic chair pose is often done with your arms stretching straight up, but any extended angle will be effective. Experiment to find the best one for you.

Benefit: To strengthen the legs, hips, back and shoulders, stimulating the bones of your pelvis, spine and legs, and to practice precise alignment

Props: None

Finer Points

- Pay special attention to the alignment of your knees and spine in this pose.
- Align your head with the rest of the spine as best you can.

Instructions

1. Stand with your feet hip-width apart and parallel to one another.
2. Press down through the four corners of each foot.
3. Bend your knees, tracking them over the second or third toes. Start with a slight bend, and increase it when you are ready.
4. Bend forward from your hips, keeping the spine long and strong and your neck in line with the rest of the spine. Do not push your chin forward.

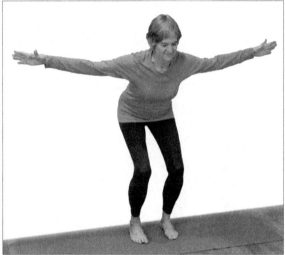

5. Isometrically push your thighs and sitting bones apart, then lengthen your tailbone and lift your abdomen and pelvic floor, all without rounding your spine.
6. Extend your arms out to the sides, squeezing your shoulder blades toward the spine.
7. Create the stabilizing and expanding energies in all parts of the body to stimulate the bones with compression and tensile stress.
8. Hold the pose as long as you can, breathing steadily.
9. When you're ready, return to standing tall.

This pose especially targets the hips and lower back, which are the locations the DEXA scan measures for bone density.

Reflections

- Can you avoid spinal flexion in this pose?
- Do you feel the stabilizing and expanding energies both working in this pose?

Dynamic Balancing

Dynamic balancing provides a playful chance to challenge your stability while moving.

Benefit: To simulate balance challenges in daily life

Props: A yoga mat and wall or chair (optional)

Finer Points

- Focus your attention on the standing leg more than the moving leg.
- Don't worry about what you look like!

Instructions

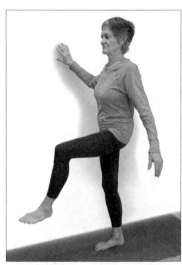

There are two variations to explore: one with your suspended leg swinging forward and backward, and the other swinging randomly. Experiment with both variations to challenge your balance in different ways.

Variation 1: One leg swinging

1. Stand while touching a wall or a chair back, if needed. Alternatively, you can stand away from the wall.
2. Starting with your feet somewhat wide apart, shift your weight to one leg, then lift the other and swing it gently forward and back. Try different speeds.
3. Focus your gaze on something straight in front of you and engage your core to stabilize your balance.
4. Bring the lifted leg down and repeat the movements on the other side.

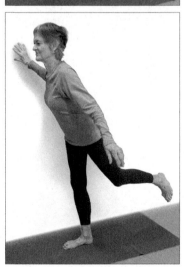

Variation 2: Side-stepping

1. Move away from the wall and stand facing into the room with your feet several inches apart so you can easily move side to side.
2. Take a wide step to the left with your left foot and lift your right foot off the ground.
3. Move your right leg in the air playfully to challenge your balance for a few seconds.

4. Lower the right foot into another wide side step, this time to the right.

5. Shift your weight onto your right foot and lift your left foot off the ground.

6. Move your left leg in the air playfully to challenge your balance for a few seconds.

7. Lower the left foot.

8. Repeat this pattern, varying the distance and the speed. Focus on how you find and sustain your balance on one leg.

9. Continue for as long as you wish, moving the lifted leg playfully in the air to challenge yourself.

Reflections

- Is one of your legs more reliable for balance than the other?

- Can you feel your coordination improving over time as you practice this exercise?

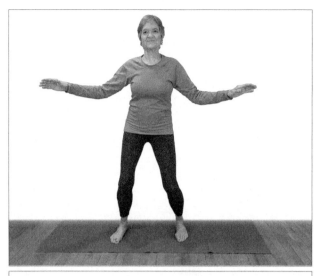

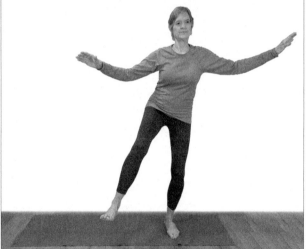

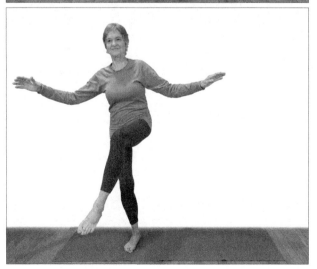

Chapter 7. Supine Series

I encourage everyone to practice this sequence of mat poses for warm-up daily. It takes about fifteen minutes and includes fundamental actions for the hips, abdominal muscles, spine and legs. These poses are all done while lying on your back.

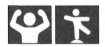

Pelvic Tilt

The pelvic tilt is a foundational movement that helps create awareness and stability in your lower back and pelvis. It's a good beginning to this supine series of exercises because we'll refer to it many times in the poses to come.

Benefit: To develop awareness of easeful movement in the lower back and pelvis

Props: A yoga mat and blanket (optional)

Finer Points

- Keep your hips on the mat as you do this movement.
- As you practice this over time, notice and enjoy the subtle sensations in your lower back, hips and abdomen.

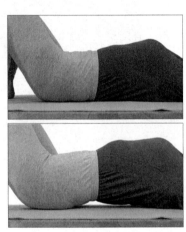

Instructions

1. Lie on your back with your knees bent and feet flat on the mat, with a folded blanket under your pelvis for comfort.
2. Press your lower back toward the floor using your abdominal muscles. Notice that your pelvis will tilt in response, with its top moving back and down and the sitting bones tilting upward into a posterior tilt of the pelvis.
3. For the anterior tilt, push your sitting bones down and lift your waistline away from the floor using your lower back muscles.
4. Practice moving from one tilt to the other as smoothly as you can.
5. Try inhaling with the anterior tilt and exhaling with the posterior tilt.
6. Find a place between the posterior and anterior tilts, and that's your neutral pelvis.

Reflections

- Which is more natural to you, the anterior or posterior tilt?
- As you become more adept at this movement, can you do it with minimal effort and maximum fluidity?

One Knee to Chest

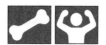

Drawing your knees to your chest, one at a time, is a safe way to practice flexion of the hips, as it loosens those joints for the poses to come. The leg movement also provides gentle strengthening for the stomach muscles while the spine remains in a neutral, supported position.

Benefit: To experience hip and thigh movement with abdominal support and without spinal flexion

Props: A yoga mat and blanket (optional)

Finer Points

- Notice the stability of your pelvis as your legs do this large movement.

Instructions

1. Lie on your back with your knees bent and feet flat on the mat, with a folded blanket under your pelvis for comfort.
2. Contract your abdominal muscles below the waist to stabilize your pelvis and lower back. Do this without changing your neutral pelvic tilt.
3. Bring one knee toward your chest and straighten the other leg on the mat.
4. Switch legs, taking care to maintain the engagement of your core muscles.
5. Alternate legs this way at a moderate pace as many times as you wish.
6. When you're ready, rest with your feet flat on the mat and take some deep breaths.

Reflections

- How does core strength support your torso while you move your legs in this way?
- How can you continue breathing smoothly while doing this exercise?

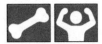

Abdominal Twist

Jathara Parivartanasana

jah-TUH-ruh pah-ree-var-tuh-NAH-suh-nuh

The support of the floor in this twisting exercise ensures the spine stays neutral as the stomach muscles are doing their work. It's a safe way to strengthen the diagonally oriented abdominal muscles that are among the prime movers in twisting poses.

Benefit: To strengthen the core muscles of the spine and torso and to learn to twist with a long spine

Props: A yoga mat, block and blanket (optional)

Finer Points

- Press your shoulders into the floor while your lower body is moving.
- Relax your neck as much as possible. Try rolling it from side to side to avoid clenching it.
- Create a breathing rhythm that works for you.

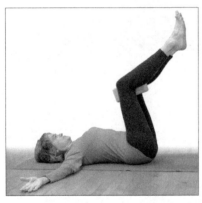

Instructions

1. Lie on your back with knees bent and arms stretched to the sides with the blanket under your pelvis or head and neck for comfort.
2. Bend your knees and place a block between them. (Use the narrow, medium or wide dimension—your choice.)
3. Squeezing the block with your knees, raise your feet as high as your knees or higher.
4. Flex your ankles and spread your toes.
5. Press your arms and shoulders into the floor to stabilize your upper torso.
6. Move your legs at a moderate pace from right to left, breathing steadily. Begin by moving a small amount and increase how far you twist when you feel ready.
7. When you are tired, come back to center, remove the block, place your feet flat, and rest.

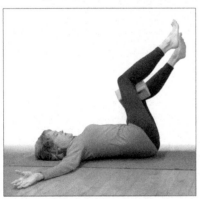

Reflections

- Are you noticing both stability and movement in this twist?
- How are you coordinating those two elements in this dynamic exercise?

Windshield Wiper

This version of the windshield wiper pose might differ from others you may have practiced, where the two knees loosely drop to one side, then the other. Here, you are active, keeping one leg in the starting position with the knee pointing upward as the other leg moves into the stretch and elongates.

Benefit: To stretch the side of the body actively

Props: A yoga mat and pillow or bolster (optional)

Finer Points

- Actively lengthen during the pose and feel the stretch all along your side. Breathe into that stretch.
- Keep your neck relaxed.

Instructions

1. Lie on your back with your knees bent, feet wide apart on the edges of the mat, and your arms stretched above your head. If this is uncomfortable for your shoulders, place a pillow or bolster above your head and rest your arms there.

2. Tilt your right knee toward your left foot, allowing your right hip to lift slightly off the floor and shift forward a bit. Your leg will rotate inward and cross your midline.

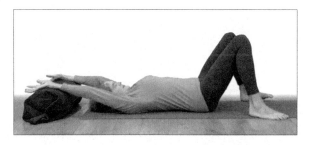

3. Allow the outside edge of your right foot to lift off the floor.

4. Leave your left knee pointing upward to stabilize your pelvis.

5. Reach your right upper leg and your right arm in opposite directions away from the hip, lengthening the entire right side of your body.

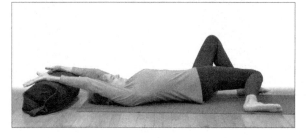

6. Feel your breath as your ribs and lungs are taking part in this pose.

7. Repeat on the other side.

8. Rest with your legs flat on the floor and feel the results in the sides of your body.

Variation

When you're working on the right side, you can grasp the right wrist with your left hand to stretch farther. And then reverse arms for the opposite side.

Reflections

- Where do you feel the most stretch: your thigh, hip, side or shoulder?
- Is there a difference between your right and left sides in this stretch?
- Is your breathing expanded by this pose?

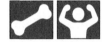

Bridge Pose

Setu Bandhasana

SAY-too bun-DAH-suh-nuh

In the bridge pose, you will lift your hips and chest away from the floor, with your feet and shoulders staying on the mat and actively pressing downward. It's a good entry-level back-bending pose.

Benefit: To stimulate the bones of the spine and hips and to improve posture by strengthening the muscles in the back of the body

Props: A yoga mat and blanket (optional)

Finer Points

- Using a blanket under your shoulders reduces the pressure on your neck. But be careful *not* to put the blanket under your neck or head since it will create too much flexion in your neck.
- Do not turn your head while in the pose.

- To stretch your shoulders more, remove the blanket and clasp your hands under your back.
- To avoid lumbar compression, pull your ribs toward your head and your pelvis toward your knees. Lengthen!

Instructions

1. Lie on your back with your knees bent, feet flat, parallel to each other, and hip-width apart. Position your arms alongside your body slightly away from your waist with your elbows bent and fingers pointing upward.

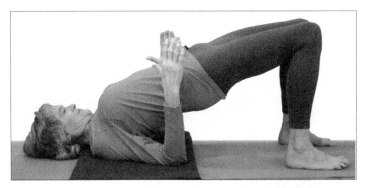

2. Lift your shoulders slightly to squeeze the blades in toward your spine, one at a time.

3. Press down through the four corners of your feet, especially the inner edges, and lift your hips with your knees pointing straight ahead toward your second and third toes.

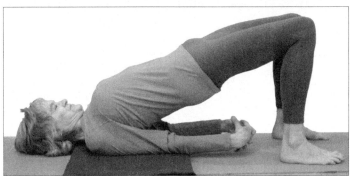

4. See if you can lift your tailbone and your chest even more.

5. As you lift higher, you will be able to tuck your shoulders under you more.

6. Remain in the pose for at least 20–30 seconds, breathing steadily.

7. When you're ready, release down to the floor and rest.

Reflections

- Can you lengthen your torso as you remain in the pose?
- Can you feel the actions of your back, hip and thigh muscles?

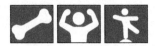

Supine Leg Stretches

Supta Padangusthasana

SOOP-tah puh-dahn-goosh-TAH-suh-nuh

This leg stretch is an important pose because it addresses stiffness in the large muscles at the backs of the legs. Lengthening these muscles helps to maintain good alignment in the pelvis and allows more freedom of movement in yoga and daily life. This pose especially helps the hips, knees and lower back.

Benefit: To stretch the hamstrings with the proper pelvic tilt, to prepare for downward-facing dog and standing poses, to stimulate the femur bones, and to feel movement at the hip joint while stabilizing the pelvis

Props: A yoga mat, belt and blanket (optional)

Finer Points

- Notice the strong isometric action in your working leg as it pushes against the belt.
- Adjust your hold on the belt to allow the working leg to fully straighten.
- Be sure to breathe naturally for the duration of the pose.

Instructions

1. Lie on your back with a blanket under you for comfort.
2. With both knees bent, practice the pelvic tilt to remember the action that creates the anterior tilt.

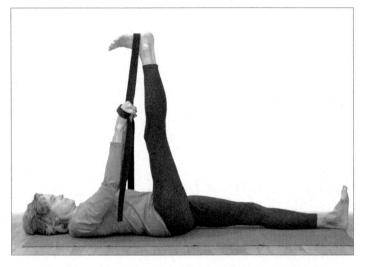

3. Lift your right knee toward your chest and loop the middle of the belt against the sole of your foot.
4. Hold the two ends of the belt with your arms gently outstretched and your shoulders on the mat, while recreating the anterior pelvic tilt.

5. Straighten your right leg, lifting your foot in the air, contracting the muscles just above your knee and adjusting your hands on the belt accordingly.

6. Press through your heel.

7. Straighten your left leg and press your thigh into the floor, which will stabilize the anterior tilt of your pelvis and make the stretch of the right leg more intense. Or keep the left leg bent if you would prefer less intensity or if you have less hip flexibility.

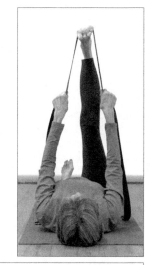

8. As you pull with the belt, push your thigh (especially at the hip area) away from your upper body, opposing the pull of the belt. There may not be any movement since you are doing an isometric contraction, but you will feel the difference. This creates a dynamic action in your hip area that stimulates the femur bone and accurately stretches your hamstring muscles.

9. The angle of the leg will vary from one person to another and will change as you practice this pose over the long term.

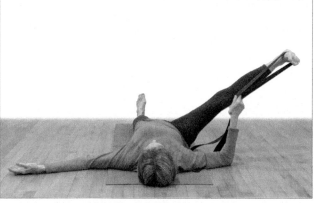

10. Hold the pose at your stretch threshold for 15–20 seconds, breathing naturally.

11. Switch both ends of the belt to your right hand and move your right leg to the side at a manageable angle for you while keeping your left hip down on the mat.

12. Engage your abdominals to stabilize your pelvis and press through both heels.

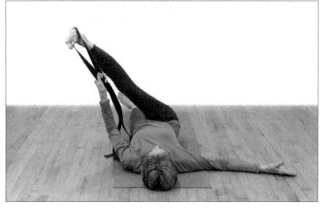

13. Hold there for 15–20 seconds, breathing naturally. Notice the abdominal work required.

14. Switch the belt to your left hand and move the right leg across your

midline at an angle that creates a stretch in your outer thigh and hip. Your right hip will be slightly off the floor.

15. Engage the muscles on all sides of your thigh.

16. Stabilize your pelvis and press through your right heel with your knee straight.

17. Hold for 15–20 seconds.

18. When you're ready, release and breathe naturally. Rest with both legs flat on the mat before changing sides.

19. Repeat the sequence with the other leg.

Reflections

- Can you keep your shoulders and neck relaxed as you do this?
- Do you feel the stabilizing and expanding energies in your legs?
- What sensations do you feel after you finish this exercise?

Chapter 8. Prone Series

The prone series is another set of poses that could be done as a ten-to-fifteen-minute practice on its own. It centers on downward-facing dog, abdominal strengtheners, and backbends, all while facing the floor.

**CHAPTER 8:
PRONE SERIES**

Cat/Cow

The cat/cow involves a gentle pattern of arching and curving your spine while on your hands and knees, which helps you feel each part of the spine as it moves.

Benefit: To move the spine in flexion and extension, exploring mobility without weight-bearing

Props: A yoga mat and blanket or pillow (optional)

Finer Points

- Find a comfortable rhythm and fluidity for this movement.

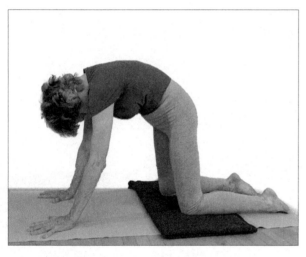

Instructions

1. Begin on your hands and knees, and move carefully and gently into spinal flexion by pushing your mid-back upward as you lengthen your tailbone and bow your head.
2. Arch your back with the midsection moving down toward the floor and the tailbone and head tilting up toward the ceiling.
3. Coordinate the movement with your breath, inhaling as you arch and exhaling as you curve.
4. Repeat 5–6 times.
5. When you're ready, release the pose.

Reflections

- What do you notice about the degree of movement in different parts of your spine (the lower, middle and upper back)?
- Is there more range of motion in this position than when you are standing up?

Balancing Table Pose

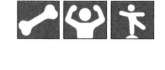

The balancing table pose is an exercise that illustrates the two principles of stability and mobility. You'll be stabilizing your lower torso and pelvis while moving your legs and arms.

Benefit: To build core strength, balance and coordination
Props: A yoga mat and blanket (optional)

Finer Points

- Maintain a neutral head position in line with the rest of your spine.
- As the arm and leg lift, maintain stability at your center.
- Play with different speeds of movement to challenge your stability.

Instructions

1. Begin on your hands and knees with the blanket under your knees for comfort.
2. Reach forward with your left hand and touch the floor lightly with your fingertips.
3. Pause and feel the engagement of your spine and shoulders, as well as your core stabilizing muscles.
4. Holding that position, stretch your right leg back and touch the floor lightly with your toes.
5. As you briefly pause, feel your hip and leg muscles as well as your core, preparing them for the next step.
6. When you're ready, lift both your left arm and your right leg, stretching them away from your center.
7. Hold that position for several breaths, then change sides, lifting your right arm and left leg.

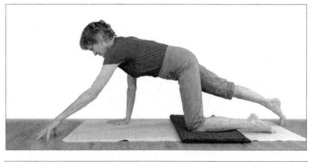
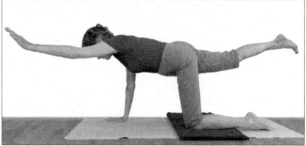

8. Keep the center of your body steady, especially your lower back and pelvis, as you move your arms and legs.
9. Lengthen both sides of your torso equally.
10. When you feel more comfortable with these movements, practice this at different speeds (slowly to build strength and quickly to build coordination and balance).

When you finish, you can remain on your hands and knees, ready for the next pose or rest in child's pose (on page 94).

Reflections

- What challenges do you feel while doing this exercise slowly? What about when you do it more quickly?
- Can you maintain a steady breathing rhythm?

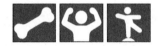

Plank Pose

Phalakasana

puh-luh-KAH-suh-nuh

Despite its simple shape, the plank pose will really help you build strength in your core and arms. The third variation also gives beneficial stimulation to the wrists.

Benefit: To build whole-body strength and stimulate the wrist bones

Props: A yoga mat

Finer Points

- Check that your ribs are in line with your shoulders, not higher or lower than them.
- Lift your pelvis and maintain its neutral tilt.
- Stretch your legs back, pressing through your heels.

Instructions

There are three progressive variations: one using forearms and knees as your foundation, the next using forearms and toes, and the last using your hands and toes. You will build strength incrementally as you progress from one variation to the next.

Variation 1: Forearm plank with knees on the mat

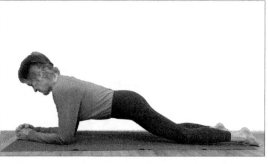

1. Begin on your hands and knees, then bring your forearms to the floor with your elbows under your shoulders, and lower your pelvis to the floor with your legs outstretched.

2. Clasp your hands and point your toes.

3. Press your forearms into the floor, so your chest lifts up and forward.

4. Lift your pelvis with your knees remaining on the mat while you look straight down at the mat.

5. Feel where strength is required and continue to breathe steadily.

6. Hold this position for 15–30 seconds.

7. When you're ready, lower your body to the floor.

8. Repeat if you wish.

Variation 2: Forearm plank with legs straight

1. Continuing from variation 1, bring the balls of your feet onto the mat, raise your heels, and straighten your knees.

2. Squeeze your shoulder blades toward your spine to support your upper back and lift your chest, pulling it forward and away from your legs. Be careful not to let your chest sag.

3. Lift your pelvis off the floor, bringing it just high enough to be in line with your ribs and shoulders, not higher or lower. There should be a straight line from your shoulders to your heels, and your weight should be on your forearms and toes.

4. Look straight down at your hands, with the back of your head at about the same level as your shoulders.

5. Hold steady and breathe for 15–30 seconds.

6. When you're ready, lower your body to the floor.

Variation 3: Full arm plank

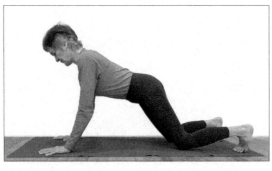

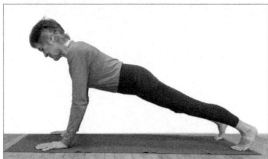

1. Begin on your hands and knees on the mat. Place your hands shoulder-width apart and rotate them slightly outward. Your index fingers should point straight ahead.
2. Rotate your upper arms forward.
3. Feel your palms evenly pressing down into the mat, including your fingertips.
4. Walk your knees back a few inches.
5. Lift your heels in the air with the balls of your feet pressing into the mat.
6. Keeping your arms and shoulders steady and strong, lift your knees to make one long line from your head to your heels.
7. Hold this pose as you breathe steadily for 15–20 seconds.
8. When you're ready, lower your body to the floor.

Reflections

- Do you feel your body strongly connected from your head to your toes?
- Can you maintain the stabilizing and expanding energies in the pose?
- Have a friend observe you and give you tips. What part of your body is too high? Too low? The goal is to have a straight line from the crown of your head to your hips or heels, depending on which variation you are doing.

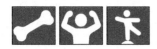

Downward-Facing Dog

Adho Mukha Svanasana

ah-doh moo-kah shvah-NAH-suh-nuh

Downward-facing dog is a well-known yoga pose in which your weight is on your hands and feet, and your hips are lifted strongly to create an inverted "V" shape. Though the outward shape is deceptively simple, there are many elements to it.

Benefit: To build strength and flexibility in the shoulders, spine and legs and to stimulate the wrist bones

Props: A yoga mat and wall

Finer Points

- The first priority is to create the anterior tilt of the pelvis. If your legs don't allow that, bend your knees and gradually work to straighten them over time.
- The second priority is to elongate your spine, avoiding flexion (or rounding).
- If your wrists bother you, keep your weight forward toward your fingers, pressing them down. You can also add a small pad (like a rolled washcloth) under your wrists.
- Keep your knees tracking properly straight ahead.

Instructions

There are two variations to choose from: one standing and the other on hands and feet. The first will work on the pelvic tilt without weight on the hands, while the latter challenges you to find a neutral tilt while both your hands and feet are bearing weight.

Variation 1: Hands on a wall

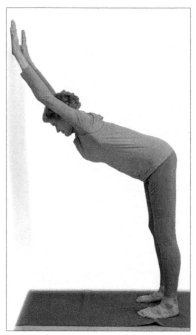

1. Stand facing a wall, and place your hands at eye level on it, shoulder-width apart.
2. Walk your feet back, while straightening your arms.
3. Reach your hips back, creating the anterior tilt of your pelvis. Bend your knees if that is helpful.
4. As you put weight on your arms, rotate the upper arms to face your biceps upward.
5. Continuously stretch through your sitting bones with strong stabilizing and expanding energies.
6. Hold the pose, breathing fully for 15–20 seconds.
7. When you're ready, step toward the wall and return to standing.

Variation 2: The full pose

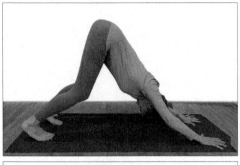

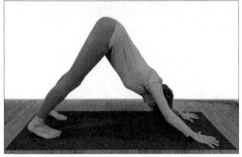

1. Begin on your hands and knees, then move your knees back a few inches.
2. Prepare your arms for weight-bearing by rotating your upper arms so your biceps turn slightly forward and rotate your hands to point your index fingers forward as well. Check that your hands are shoulder-width apart. Press your fingertips down.
3. Bring the balls of your feet onto the mat, raise your heels, and gently arch your back.
4. Lift your knees off the floor as you inhale, and exhale as you pull your pelvis up and back, keeping your knees bent at first. Lift your sitting bones to avoid rounding your spine.
5. When you're ready, straighten one leg at a time, pressing the heel down and feeling the stretch along the back of your leg.
6. If possible, straighten both legs, pushing your knees back, lifting your sitting bones, and stretching your heels downward.
7. Feel your hands, continuing to press your fingertips down to avoid excess pressure on your wrists.
8. Contract your arm muscles from your wrists into your shoulders to maintain strength.
9. Breathe deeply to maintain your energy as you hold the pose for 20–30 seconds.
10. Exhale as you come down to rest.

It's very common to do child's pose after this one. (See "Child's Pose" on page 94.)

Reflections

- Do you feel your pelvis actively reaching up?
- Can you feel how bending your knees helps to elongate your spine?
- Can you be patient with yourself as you work toward strength and flexibility in this pose?

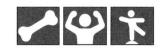

Cobra Pose

Bhujangasana

boo-jang-GAH-suh-nuh

In the cobra pose, you start by lying face down, and then your spine lengthens and arches, pulling forward and elongating the torso.

Benefit: To strengthen the upper back, spinal vertebrae, shoulders, arms and wrists

Props: A yoga mat

Finer Points

- Spread the effort throughout the length of your spine as you pull your chest forward away from your pelvis.
- Avoid overusing your arms or underusing your spine.
- If your lower back feels pinched, stay closer to the floor, pulling your chest forward away from your hips while extending your legs and hips back. Use the expanding energy to elongate your whole body.

Instructions

There are two variations: one with your hands forward, and the other with your hands placed farther back and wider apart. The first variation requires less flexibility in your spine, while the second lifts you higher into the pose.

Variation 1: Hands forward

1. Lie face down on your mat and place your elbows on the floor under your shoulders with your chest lifted away from the floor. Point your hands straight ahead on the mat.
2. Squeeze your shoulder blades together and contract the muscles of your spine, establishing the stabilizing energy.
3. Elongate through your whole body, bringing your chest forward and your legs back with the expanding energy.
4. One leg at a time, lift and turn the front of the leg in toward the midline to widen the back of the pelvis, then stretch your leg and lower it to the floor. Repeat with the other leg.

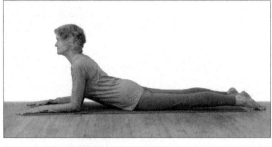

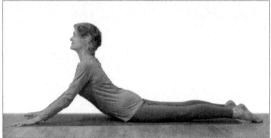

This preparation will lengthen your lower back and hips.

5. Maintaining your shoulder position, press your hands down and lift your elbows off the floor, arching your upper back. Reach your head upward, keeping your neck long on all sides. Gaze upward if your neck allows. Your arms can remain slightly bent or straightened.

6. Stay in the pose for 15–30 seconds, continuing to support it with the stabilizing and expanding energies.

7. Keep breathing into the front, back and sides of your chest.

8. Return to a resting position with your head to one side.

Variation 2: The full pose

1. Beginning with your forehead on the floor, stretch your legs and point your toes.

2. Place your hands to the sides of your shoulders.

3. Squeeze your shoulder blades toward the spine and pull your shoulders away from your ears.

4. Activate your legs and buttocks, lengthening them behind you.

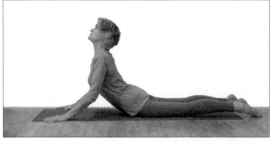

5. Lift your torso, leading with your head, and reaching up and out from your pelvis through the top of your head.

6. Press down gently with your hands, but avoid causing compression in your lower back, which can come from overusing your arms or rising too far.

7. Attempt to activate each section of your spine to make this arching shape.

8. Breathe and expand for 15–30 seconds, then come back down to rest.

9. Repeat if you wish.

Reflections

- Can you find the right height of this pose for you, where your spine is working strongly without discomfort and you feel a stretch in your abdomen?
- How many repetitions of this pose feels right for you?

Locust Pose

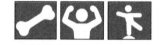

Salabhasana (or Shalabhasana)

shuh-luh-BAH-suh-nuh

With the locust pose, you'll lift from the floor in a similar shape to the cobra pose, but without your arms pressing down. Imagine that you're flying!

Benefit: To strengthen all muscles in the back of the body and to stimulate the vertebrae and pelvic bones

Props: A yoga mat and blanket

Finer Points

- If you have discomfort in your lower back, stay closer to the floor and contract your buttocks and stomach muscles more strongly. The locust pose is for strength, not range of motion. Lifting just a small amount yields its benefits.

Instructions

1. Lie face down on the mat with the blanket under your pelvis, legs extended, arms out to the sides, and palms down.
2. Feel your breath expand the back of your body and elongate from your hips to your feet.
3. Squeeze your shoulder blades toward your spine and slightly down toward your hips.
4. Contract the muscles around your spine, creating the stabilizing energy.
5. Lift your arms and shoulders away from the floor, then your head, followed by your legs. Try to bring your thighs off the floor too.
6. Extend out from the center of your body through your legs, arms and head, using the expanding energy.

7. Continue to breathe steadily, holding the pose as long as you can. Then release.

8. Feel your breath expand the back of your body again.

9. Repeat if you wish.

It's very common to do child's pose after this one. (See "Child's Pose" on page 94.)

Reflections

• Do you feel your entire back working strongly?

• Does the expanding energy help to avoid lower back compression?

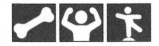

Low Lunge Pose with Backbend

Anjaneyasana

ahn-jah-nay-AH-suh-nuh

When you do a low lunge with a backbend, one leg is forward and the other back, while you add a backbend. You can progress into it gradually, stopping at any point.

Benefit: To strengthen the spine and thighs, stretch the hips, and improve balance

Props: A yoga mat, blanket and two blocks

Finer Points

• Use the stabilizing and expanding energies to maintain full strength in your pelvis and legs for stability.

• Stretch out from the pelvis with your spine, legs and arms.

• If you start to lose your balance in the third variation, bring your hands to the front of your thigh or to the blocks.

Instructions

There are three variations for this pose. The first uses the blocks to help you establish your balance while looking straight ahead. The second adds a spinal extension (arch) and increased hip stretch as you look upward, while still touching the blocks. The third brings your arms behind as you arch your back, making it more challenging to maintain your balance.

Variation 1: Establish balance

1. Begin on your hands and knees, with your knees on the blanket and your hands on the blocks in front of you at their highest dimension.
2. Step forward with your right foot between the blocks and your toes pointing forward.
3. Move your left knee back a few inches, bring the ball of your left foot onto the mat and raise your heel for stability.
4. Move the blocks back near your hips.
5. Extend your spine up and out of your pelvis.
6. Contract the muscles of your pelvis and legs with stabilizing energy.
7. Lengthen your tailbone and lift your torso as much as possible. Expand your entire body, especially your spine and back leg.
8. Press your hands down into the blocks for help with balance.
9. Hold the pose with confidence and strength, breathing normally.
10. When you're ready, release the pose.
11. Repeat on the other side.

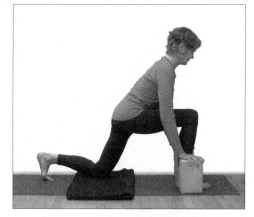

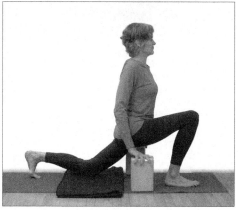

Variation 2: Increase hip flexibility

1. Continuing from variation 1, move your pelvis a bit forward toward your front foot. You'll notice a stronger stretch in the hip and thigh of your back leg.
2. Press down into the blocks with your hands and lift your chest forward and up.
3. While looking upward, maintain a safe and comfortable range of motion in your neck. (For a refresher, see "Neck Extension" on page 54.)
4. Hold the pose with steady strength and expansion throughout your body.

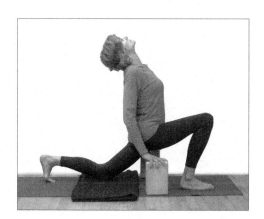

5. When you're ready, return to looking straight ahead.

6. Switch legs and repeat on the other side.

Variation 3: Improve spinal strength and balance

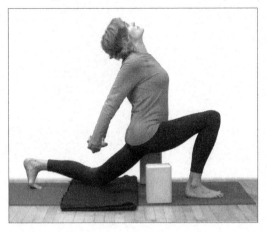

1. After completing variations 1 and 2, let go of the blocks and stretch your arms out to the side or clasp your hands behind your back.

2. Lift your spine up and out of your pelvis, maintaining your balance as you look upward.

3. Stay in the pose for 15–30 seconds.

4. When you're ready, release the pose.

5. Switch legs and repeat on the other side.

Reflections

- Do you feel your core strongly even as you look upward?

- What do you feel in your hips and spine after doing this pose?

Child's Pose

Balasana

bah-LAH-suh-nuh

Child's pose is a well-known resting yoga pose. In these variations, we use extra props to ensure safe spinal alignment and protection from possible discomfort in the knees as we rest the spine.

Benefit: To stimulate the front part of the vertebrae and to release the spine and rest after any vigorous practice

Props: A yoga mat, chair, bolster, block and two or three blankets or towels

Finer Points

- If you have knee pain in this pose, practice it with two chairs. While sitting in a chair with your legs wide apart, bend forward at your hips to rest your arms and head on the second chair.

- Increase your relaxation by breathing slowly and expansively. You can intentionally breathe into different parts of your body to see what feels best.

Instructions

There are three variations for this pose, each using a different prop for upper body support: either a chair, a bolster or a block. Choose which variation you want to do based on the flexibility of your hips. A higher prop requires less flexibility.

> **Caution:** This is a forward bend, so take care to elongate your spine, allowing only a very small amount of rounding as you fold forward with your upper body, flexing at your hips.

Variation 1: With your arms and head resting on a chair seat

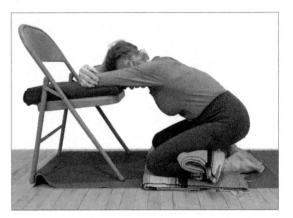

1. Place a chair at the short end of your mat with the seat facing the middle and one folded blanket on it. Then set another folded blanket on the mat for your knees.
2. Kneel on the mat facing the chair.
3. Adjust your position so your feet are halfway off the back edge of the blanket to ease the pressure on your ankles.
4. Spread your knees apart about 12–16″.
5. Tuck a folded or rolled blanket behind your knees as a spacer and cushion.
6. Move your hips back toward your feet, as if sitting on your heels, and your torso forward toward the chair seat.
7. Rest your arms and head on the chair, finding a comfortable position.
8. Breathe slowly and deeply for several minutes, allowing your spine and legs to relax.
9. Come up when you are ready.

Variation 2: With your torso resting on a bolster

1. Kneel on a folded blanket with your knees wide apart and your big toes touching.
2. Set a bolster lengthwise in front of you and place a block under it toward the far end, about two-thirds away from

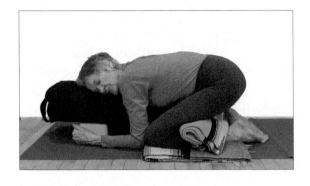

you. The block should be perpendicular to the bolster and at a comfortable height.

3. Tuck a folded or rolled blanket behind your knees as a spacer and cushion.

4. Move your hips back toward your feet, as if sitting on your heels, and pull the bolster toward you to support your entire torso.

5. Lower yourself onto the bolster with your hips elongating toward your heels.

6. Add another folded blanket or towel on top of the bolster if needed for comfort and height.

7. Turn your head to one side and place your forearms on the floor.

8. Settle into the pose, breathing slowly and deeply for several minutes.

9. Come up when you are ready.

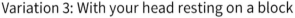

Variation 3: With your head resting on a block

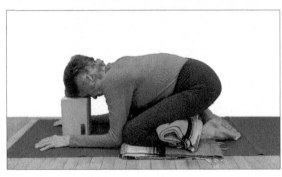

1. Kneel on a folded blanket with your knees wide apart and big toes touching.

2. Set a block in front of you to support your head when you're in the pose.

3. Adjust your position so your feet are halfway off the back edge of the blanket to ease the pressure on your ankles.

4. Tuck a rolled or folded blanket behind your knees as a spacer and cushion.

5. Move your hips back, as if sitting on your heels.

6. Lengthen your torso and rest your forehead on the block, adjusting its height to minimize the rounding of your spine.

7. Find a comfortable position for your arms.

8. Relax into the pose, breathing deeply and exhaling fully for several minutes.

9. Come up when you are ready.

Reflections

- What do you feel in your back, hips, knees and ankles in this pose?
- Does resting your head on a support and focusing on your breath feel relaxing to you?

Chapter 9. Chair Series

This short series requires the use of a chair to address the essential actions of the spine and hips. These backbends, twists and hip stretches can be done as a warm-up or on their own when your time is limited.

CHAPTER 9
CHAIR SERIES

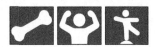

Seated Spinal Arch

The seated spinal arch is a simple back strengthener that can be done anytime during your day, especially if your work involves extended time in a chair.

Benefit: To strengthen the spinal muscles

Props: A chair and blanket (optional)

Finer Points

- Simultaneously root down into your sitting bones and reach up with your chest and head.
- Notice which parts of your spine move more easily and which parts feel less mobile.

Instructions

1. Sit on the chair as far forward on the seat as possible with a folded blanket under you for comfort.
2. With your hands, hold the sides of the seat behind you.
3. Strongly engage the muscles in your upper back, squeezing your shoulder blades together and reaching your chest up and forward.
4. As much as possible, lift the front of your ribs.
5. Arch your neck carefully, following the instructions for the "Neck Extension" on page 54.
6. Take several deep breaths, extending upward throughout your whole upper body.
7. Release and look straight ahead, bringing your hands to your thighs.

Reflections

- Can you lift your ribs up and away from your pelvis in this pose?
- Do you feel any stretching in your abdomen or chest?

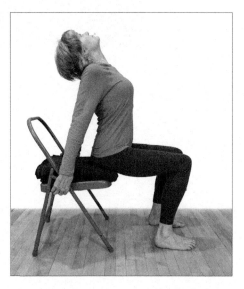

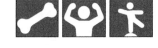

Seated Twist

When you twist while sitting in a chair, you'll have a good opportunity to isolate the action to your spine, thanks to the contact with the chair. And like the previous pose, it's an easy one to use as a refreshing movement break while working at your desk.

Benefit: To twist the spine with the hips and legs stable, stimulating the vertebrae and hips

Props: A chair without arms and a block (optional)

Finer Points

- Use a block between your knees to provide more stability in your pelvis.
- Keep your head over your pelvis, avoiding any sideways bending in your spine.
- Keep your chest broad, squeezing your shoulder blades together.
- Lengthen your spine as you inhale and twist slightly more as you exhale.

Instructions

There are two variations. The first is with your legs parallel, and the next with your legs crossed. Having your legs parallel is a great way to stabilize the pelvis. When you cross your legs in the second variation, you'll get extra bone stimulation in your hips.

Variation 1: Legs parallel

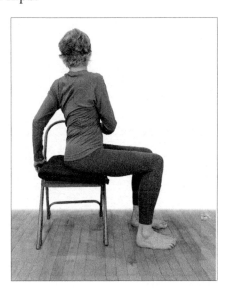

1. Sit sideways in the chair with your left side toward the back of the chair.
2. Place your feet hip-width apart and parallel, knees over the ankles.
3. Point your toes and knees straight ahead.
4. Inhale while lifting your spine.
5. Exhale while twisting from the waist up, toward the back of the chair. Use your arms on the back of the chair to enhance the twist, but perform most of the action with your spinal and abdominal muscles, keeping your pelvis steady.

6. Breathe normally as you hold the pose for 15–30 seconds.

7. When you're ready, release the pose.

8. To repeat on the other side, sit with your right side toward the back of the chair.

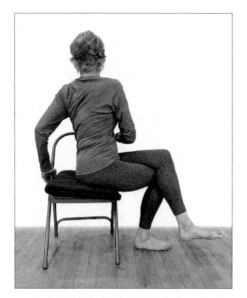

Variation 2: Legs crossed

For this variation, repeat the actions listed above, but start by sitting sideways on your chair with your left side toward its back and then cross your left leg over the right.

Reflections

- What do you feel in each part of your spine during this twist (in your mid-back, upper back, and neck)?

- How does your breathing feel different while twisting, as compared to sitting in a neutral forward-facing position?

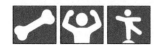

Ankle to Knee

The ankle to knee pose is similar to the way some people sit casually, with one ankle placed on the opposite knee, but we add more specific actions to it to increase its benefit.

Benefit: To stimulate the hip bones and stretch the hip muscles

Props: A chair and blanket (optional)

Finer Points

- Check that the knee and foot of the supporting leg point straight ahead.

- Notice how the little details accentuate the stretch.

Instructions

1. Sitting in the chair with a folded blanket under you for comfort, reach under one upper thigh with your hands and pull the muscles back and to the side.

2. Repeat on the other leg. This manual adjustment will initiate the anterior pelvic tilt. Notice how this helps you to sit tall.

3. While maintaining your pelvic tilt as much as possible, place your right ankle across your left knee. If the tilt disappears, re-establish it after your ankle is in place.

4. Place your right hand on the outside of the right knee and your left hand on the sole of your right foot. Press in with both hands as you internally push your thighs away from each other, as in "Outer Thigh Strengthening" on page 52. You'll feel a strong sensation on the outside of your right hip.

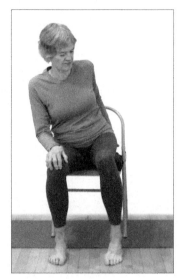

5. If you want to stretch even more, lean forward slightly, flexing your hips without rounding your spine, and lengthen your spine upward.

6. Keep all the actions going: establishing hip flexion without spinal flexion, pressing the thighs apart, and lengthening up and out through your torso.

7. Hold for 15–30 seconds, then release.

8. Repeat on the other side.

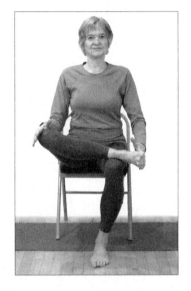

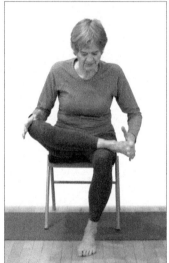

Reflections

- Where is the strongest sensation for you: the inner thigh, the outer thigh or the hip joint?
- Can you avoid spinal flexion as you bend forward over your legs?

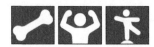

Camel Pose

Ustrasana

oosh-TRAH-suh-nuh

In camel pose, you are on your knees and lower legs, then you lift your spine into a backbend with your hands touching a support.

Benefit: To strengthen the spine in a back-bending pose, stimulating the vertebrae and improving posture

Props: A yoga mat, blanket, chair and bolster

Finer Points

- If you feel any compression or discomfort in your lower back, lengthen your tailbone and lift your ribs more.
- Avoid dropping your head back or holding your breath. In my classes, I instruct students to sing a little song to be sure their throat is open.

Instructions

There are four variations of the camel pose. The first uses a chair, the next, a bolster, the third, your heels, and the last is the full pose. As you progress through these variations, you will develop increasing flexibility in your spine.

Variation 1: Reaching for the chair

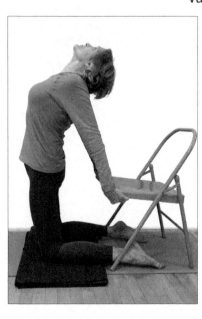

1. Place a folded blanket on the mat in front of a chair.
2. Kneel on the blanket, facing away from the chair seat.
3. Point your lower legs and feet behind you, slightly under the chair, with your ankles in line with your knees.
4. Lean forward slightly to spread your upper thighs apart, then come upright again as you lengthen your tailbone. These two actions protect and align your lower back and pelvis.
5. Use your strength to stabilize your legs and hips, then lift your spine up and out of your pelvis.
6. Pull your shoulders back and lift your chest as much as possible while remaining grounded through your legs and pelvis.

7. Reach back with one hand to grip the side of the chair seat, and then do the same with the other hand. The next time you do this pose, reverse which hand reaches back first.

8. Perform the "Neck Extension" from page 54, reaching your head up and back with support on all sides of your neck.

9. Lift your chest again as much as possible as you breathe for 15–30 seconds.

10. Return to an upright position with your spine and head, then rest in any position of your choice.

Variation 2: Reaching for the bolster

1. Place a folded blanket on the mat and kneel on it.

2. Point your lower legs and feet behind you, with your ankles in line with your knees.

3. Place the bolster across the backs of your ankles.

4. Lean forward slightly to spread your upper thighs apart, then come upright again as you lengthen your tailbone. These two actions protect and align your lower back and pelvis.

5. Use your strength to stabilize your legs and hips, then lift your spine up and out of your pelvis.

6. Pull your shoulders back and lift your chest as much as possible while remaining grounded through your legs and pelvis.

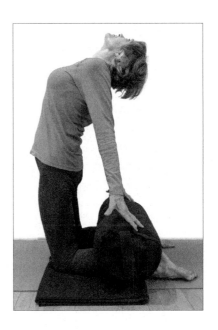

7. Reach back with one hand to place it on the bolster, and then do the same with the other hand. The next time you do this pose, reverse which hand reaches back first.

8. Perform the "Neck Extension" from page 54, reaching your head up and back with support on all sides of your neck.

9. Lift your chest again as much as possible as you breathe for 15–30 seconds.

10. Return to an upright position with your spine and head, then rest in any position of your choice.

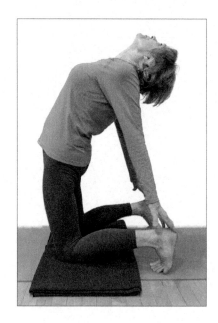

Variation 3: Reaching for your heels

1. Place a folded blanket on the mat and kneel on it.
2. Point your lower legs and feet behind you, with your ankles in line with your knees.
3. Lift your heels in the air with the balls of your feet pressing into the mat.
4. Lean forward slightly to spread your upper thighs apart, then come upright again as you lengthen your tailbone. These two actions protect and align your lower back and pelvis.
5. Use your strength to stabilize your legs and hips, then lift your spine up and out of your pelvis.
6. Pull your shoulders back and lift your chest as much as possible while remaining grounded through your legs and pelvis.
7. Reach back with one hand to place it on your heel, and then do the same with the other hand. The next time you do this pose, reverse which hand reaches back first.
8. Perform the "Neck Extension" from page 54, reaching your head up and back with support on all sides of your neck.
9. Lift your chest again as much as possible as you breathe for 15–30 seconds.
10. Return to an upright position with your spine and head, then rest in any position of your choice.

Variation 4: Toes pointed

1. Place a folded blanket on the mat and kneel on it.
2. Point your lower legs and feet behind you, with your ankles in line with your knees.
3. Point your toes toward the short end of the mat. This will result in the tops of your feet resting on it.
4. Lean forward slightly to spread your upper thighs apart, then come upright again as you lengthen your tailbone. These two actions protect and align your lower back and pelvis.

5. Use your strength to stabilize your legs and hips, then lift your spine up and out of your pelvis.

6. Pull your shoulders back and lift your chest as much as possible while remaining grounded through your legs and pelvis.

7. Reach back with one hand to place it on your heel, and then do the same with the other hand. The next time you do this pose, reverse which hand reaches back first.

8. Perform the "Neck Extension" from page 54, reaching your head up and back with support on all sides of your neck.

9. Lift your chest again as much as possible as you breathe for 15–30 seconds.

10. Return to an upright position with your spine and head, then rest in any position of your choice.

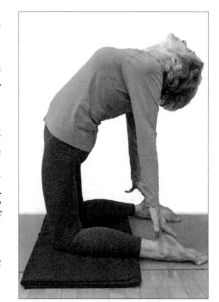

Reflections

- As you press your lower legs downward, can you lift your chest more?
- Do you feel some stretch in your arms in this pose?

Garland Pose

Malasana

mah-LAH-suh-nuh

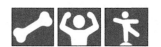

This variation of garland pose is done while seated in a chair, with your legs wide apart and your knees and feet carefully aligned. You'll fold forward from the hips, keeping your spine long.

Benefit: To stretch the inner thighs and the back of the torso, opening the hips for ease in getting down to the floor and back up again; to practice knee tracking in a wide-leg position

Props: A chair and two blocks

Finer Points

- If you have osteopenia or osteoporosis, be extra careful to keep your spine elongated rather than rounding forward.

- Push your knees away from each other (as in "Outer Thigh Strengthening" on page 52) and make sure to point them toward the second and third toes.

Instructions

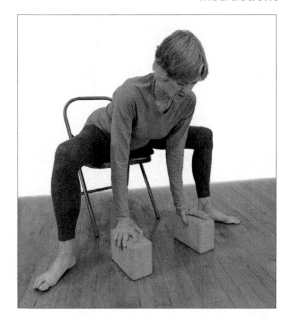

1. Sit on the chair with the blocks on the floor in front of you at a comfortable height.
2. Widen your legs apart as far as you can with the knees and feet pointing at the same angle to each side. You should be able to feel the four corners of your feet.
3. Inhale while lifting your spine up and out of your pelvis and angle your torso forward with hip flexion, but without spinal flexion. (Remember to maintain a neutral pelvis, as on page 46.) You can push your knees apart with your hands to align them over your ankles.
4. Place your hands on the blocks and continue to elongate through the top of your head. If possible, stack the two blocks together and rest your head on them, putting your hands on the floor.
5. Breathe for 15–30 seconds, noticing where you feel the strength and stretch in this pose.
6. When you're ready, return to sitting upright.

Reflections

- Do you feel the stretch in your inner thighs, hips and lower back in this pose?
- Do your knees tend to turn in toward the midline as you lean your torso forward? If so, can you keep them wide apart?

Chapter 10. Wrist and Hand Series

It's important to maintain healthy wrists, since we may need to catch ourselves from a fall with our hands and don't want to break anything when we do. These four exercises can be done anytime during your day, especially if you spend extensive time at a computer. You can also add them to your daily yoga practice to help prepare the hands and wrists for weight-bearing poses.

Wrist Extension

These two stretches are for the palm side of your wrists and forearms. For anyone who works with their hands (don't we all?), stretching this muscle group helps to maintain your range of motion and prevent wrist injuries.

Benefit: To stretch the flexor muscles of the wrists and stimulate the bones

Props: None

Finer Points

- Maintain an upright posture with your spine, pulling your shoulders back as you do this stretch.
- Continue to breathe normally and avoid creating tension in your neck.

Instructions

There are two variations of equal merit, so be sure to practice them both. You can do them either sitting or standing, whichever you prefer.

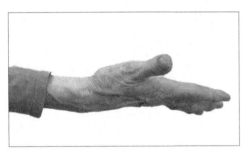

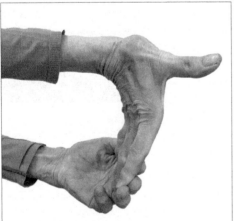

Variation 1: Lower arm palm up

1. From a comfortable position, extend your right arm in front of you with your palm facing up.
2. Using your left hand, bend your right wrist to angle the palm and fingers downward. Your right palm will face away from you.
3. Straighten your right arm.
4. Hold for 15–20 seconds.
5. When you're ready, release and give your hands a shake.
6. Repeat on the other side.

Variation 2: Lower arm palm down

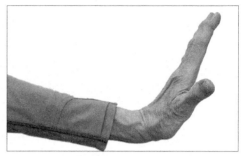

1. From a comfortable position, extend your left arm in front of you with your palm facing down.
2. Bend your wrist to point your fingers upward with your palm straight forward as if signaling to "stop."
3. Using your right hand, pull the fingers of your left hand back for a more intense extension of your wrist.
4. Keep your left elbow straight as you push your left wrist forward and continue to pull the fingers back with your right hand.
5. Hold for 15–20 seconds.
6. When you're ready, release and give your hands a shake.
7. Repeat on the other side.

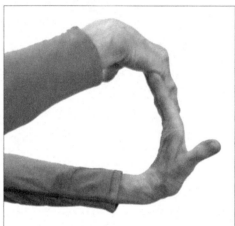

Reflections

- Do you feel a difference in sensation between these two variations?
- What activities in your daily life might lead to tension in this part of your arms?

Wrist Flexion

This wrist exercise balances the previous one, stretching the other side of the wrist and forearm by flexing it. It's particularly helpful if you are not accustomed to bearing weight on your hands, as we do in some yoga poses in this book.

Benefit: To stretch the back part of your wrists, giving tensile stress to the bones

Props: None

Finer Points

- Keeping your hands steady, try turning the inside of your elbow in toward the midline, then turning it upward. Stay with the position that feels best to you.
- Maintain an upright posture with your spine, pulling your shoulders back as you do this stretch.
- Continue to breathe normally and avoid creating tension in your neck.

Instructions

You can do this pose either sitting or standing, whichever you prefer.

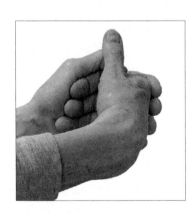

1. From a comfortable position, extend your right arm in front of you as if you are about to shake hands with someone. Curl your fingers, making a soft fist.
2. Wrap your left hand around the fist and use it to pull your palm and fingers farther into that rounded shape. Ideally, you want your wrist to create a 90-degree angle along your forearm and the back of your hand, if you can.
3. Stretch your right arm forward with your elbow straight.
4. Hold for 20–30 seconds.
5. When you're ready, change hands and repeat.

Reflections

- Do you feel the stretch in your forearm, perhaps up to your elbow?
- What activities in your daily life might lead to tension in this part of your arms?

Interlaced Twisting

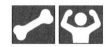

We don't usually think of our wrists as joints that twist, but with many small bones involved, we do have that range of motion. This exercise helps to keep the connective tissue and muscles healthy.

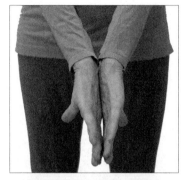

Benefit: To stretch the wrist muscles and stimulate the wrist bones

Props: None

Finer Points

- Keep your shoulders neutral and relaxed away from your ears.
- Go into each movement and position slowly and gently at first, then gradually increase the degree of twisting.

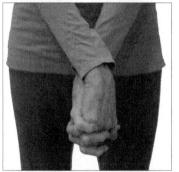

Instructions

1. Stand with your hands extended in front of you, touching their backs together.
2. Cross your right hand over the left and interlace your fingers.
3. Bend your wrists and make a side to side movement, bringing your clasped hands to the left and right several times as a warm-up.
4. Then keep your hands on one side and rotate your clasped hands to twist your wrists so your palms are parallel to the floor.

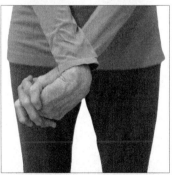

5. Hold that position for 15 seconds or so.
6. Keeping the same clasp, release the twist from step 4.
7. Shift your hands to the other side and again rotate your hands to twist your wrists so your palms are parallel to the floor.
8. Hold that position for 15 seconds or so.
9. Release your clasp and shake your hands.
10. When you're ready, repeat with the left hand on top.

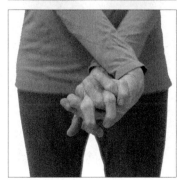

Reflections

- Can you find the appropriate degree of effort to bring to this exercise to feel a productive stretch without pain?
- Is there a noticeable difference between your two hands in this stretch?

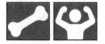

Ridgetops

Doing ridgetops brings weight to your wrist bones to stimulate them, by lifting your palms up and putting your weight on your fingers only. The stretch on the underside of your fingers will help you when weight-bearing on your hands in other poses.

Benefit: To strengthen the wrist bones and muscles and stretch the finger joints

Props: A mat

Finer Points

- Keep your shoulders neutral and relaxed away from your ears.
- At first, you may feel a strong stretch in your fingers. If it's too intense, lift your wrists only a few inches off the floor. Progress to lifting as high as possible as you gain strength and flexibility.

Instructions

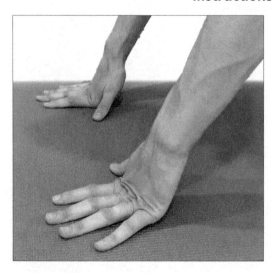

1. Begin on your hands and knees, placing your hands on the mat, shoulder-width apart and slightly angled outward toward the edges of the mat. Your index fingers should point straight ahead.
2. Lift your palms and wrists off the mat, bringing your weight forward onto your first three fingers. Your thumbs will still touch the mat lightly.
3. Feel the strength of the muscles around your wrists.
4. Practice this for 30 seconds at a time.
5. Release your hands and shake them gently.

When you feel comfortable, try increasing the weight on your fingers by doing plank pose or downward-facing dog using this hand position.

Reflections

- Does this stretch bring more awareness to the various parts of your hands?
- Is there a difference between your two hands when you do this stretch?

Chapter 11. Standing Series

The standing poses are exceptionally good for building muscular strength, balance and confidence. They strongly stimulate the bones of your spine, pelvis and thighs, helping to prevent fractures.

When your legs are spread apart, you can determine the best width for you, according to your size and flexibility. In general, a shorter distance between your feet will help your stability, and a longer distance will help you develop flexibility. I encourage you to experiment and consult with a qualified teacher if possible.

Start with the first six poses in this chapter, then add more when you are ready. Some of the poses can be practiced in pairs (as noted in the text). For example, you can do the first pose on the right side, followed by a second pose on the right side, and then do both on the left side one after the other.

Mountain Pose

Tadasana

tah-DAH-suh-nuh

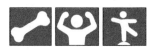

Mountain pose forms the basis of all the other standing poses, so it bears repeating. Here, we revisit the alignments that will refine all the other poses.

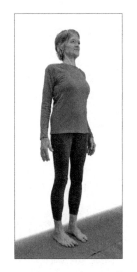

For complete instructions on how to do this pose, refer to "Mountain Pose" on page 60.

Chair Pose

Utkatasana

oot-kah-TAH-suh-nuh

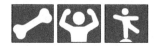

In the chair pose, you incorporate many of the skills from earlier in this book into one powerful standing pose. Notice how many of the alignments and actions you can do simultaneously.

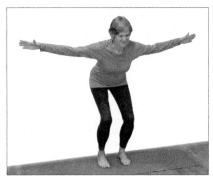

This pose is one of the most important ones you can do because it strengthens the bones of your pelvis, spine and legs. It also exemplifies hip flexion without spinal flexion.

For complete instructions on how to do this pose, refer to "Chair Pose" on page 66.

Leaning Goddess

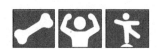

Leaning Goddess is a standing pose where your legs are wide apart with knees bent, and your upper body is leaning forward. I have added the word "leaning" to its name to distinguish it from the common version of this pose, which is done with an upright torso. This leaning version is safe for the knee and hip joints, while effectively building strength in the entire body.

Benefit: To build core strength, stretch the hips, and align the knees precisely

Props: A yoga mat, chair without arms and blanket (optional)

Finer Points

- Remember to use these fundamental actions: hip flexion without spinal flexion, the anterior tilt of your pelvis, your outer thigh strength, the four corners of your feet, and the stabilizing and expanding energies.

Instructions

There are two variations of this pose, sitting and standing. Sitting makes it easier for you to align the knees without bearing your entire body weight, so balance is not an issue. Standing requires more strength and stability.

Variation 1: Sitting

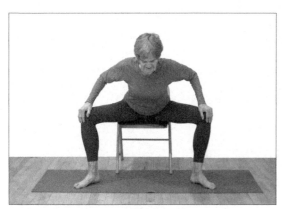
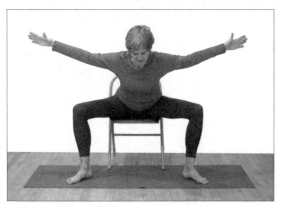

1. Sit on the front edge of the chair seat on a folded blanket for comfort, then tip your pelvis into the anterior tilt.
2. Spread your legs apart, turning your knees and feet out at the same angle.
3. Check that your knees are over your ankles and pointing toward your second and third toes.
4. Press down on all four corners of your feet.
5. Inhaling, lift your spine up and out of your pelvis and squeeze your shoulder blades toward your spine.
6. Exhaling, bend forward from the hips keeping your spine elongated.
7. Bring your hands to your knees and gently push them wider apart.
8. Then stretch your arms out to the sides. Angle your head forward, aligning with your spine, and make your neck long on all sides.

9. Energize the entire pose, elongating your spine while lifting your abdomen and pelvic floor.

10. Hold for 15–30 seconds.

11. When you're ready, release.

Variation 2: Standing

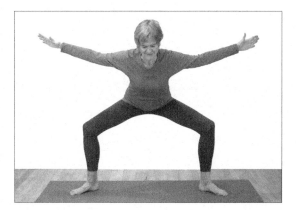

1. Stand on your mat and spread your feet about 3' apart.

2. Turn your legs out about 45 degrees, making sure that your knees and toes face the same angle.

3. Press down through the four corners of your feet.

4. Inhaling, elongate your spine up and out of your pelvis.

5. Exhaling, bend your knees and hips, leaning forward as you pull your pelvis back.

6. With your hands on your knees, push them wider apart and check that your knees are over your ankles, pointing toward the second and third toes.

7. Lift and engage your abdomen and pelvic floor without curving your spine.

8. Squeeze your shoulder blades toward your spine and stretch your arms to the sides with full extension through your fingertips.

9. Hold for 15–20 seconds, strengthening your center and expanding from there throughout your body.

10. Stand up straight and bring your feet together.

Reflections

- Which parts of your body are working most strongly in this pose?

- Can you maintain steady strength with a normal breathing rhythm as you hold this pose?

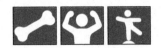

Note: Once you learn the next two poses (warrior 2 and side angle pose), they can be done as a series: completing both poses on the right first, then both on the left.

Warrior 2

Virabhadrasana 2

vee-rah-bah-DRAH-suh-nuh

Warrior 2 is done with your legs wide apart and one leg bent while the other is straight. Your spine is upright as you look to one side. In this pose, you embody strength, dignity and focus.

Benefit: To stimulate the hip and pelvic bones while building strength, confidence and balance

Props: A yoga mat and a chair or wall (optional)

Finer Points

- The width between your two feet is proportional to your height. So, taller people will need a wider stance. Experiment to determine what's best for you.
- The alignment of the bent knee is crucial in this pose. Do not allow it to turn inward. If this is difficult for you, rotate your pelvis a little more toward the bent-leg side.
- Avoid leaning your upper body toward your bent leg. Keep it over the center of your pelvis.
- Maintain strength in your back leg and arm by stretching through your fingers and pressing the outer heel of the back foot down.

Instructions

There are two variations for this pose: one with a prop for balance and the other without. Start with the first variation and, as you gain confidence in your stability, try doing the pose without assistance.

Variation 1: With a chair or wall

1. Stand facing the long side of the mat with your feet about 3′ apart. If you feel unsteady, stand with your back near a wall or place a chair in front of you so you can hold its back until you feel secure.
2. Turn your right foot and leg out to be parallel to the long edge of your mat, leaving your left foot parallel to the

short end. This will rotate your pelvis slightly to the right. From the waist up, face the long edge of the mat.

3. With your upper body vertical directly over your pelvis and turned slightly to the left, spread your arms wide, parallel to the long side of the yoga mat.

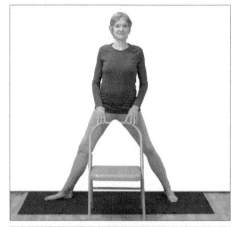

4. Squeeze your shoulder blades toward the spine, and at the same time, stretch out through your fingers, using the stabilizing and expanding energies at the same time.

5. Inhaling, elongate your spine while remaining steady on your legs.

6. Exhaling, bend your right knee, bringing it directly over your ankle, pointing toward your second and third toes.

7. Hold the pose as you turn your head to look toward your right hand.

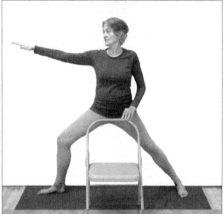

8. Remain there for 15–20 seconds, breathing steadily.

9. When you're ready, release and stand tall, returning your right leg and foot to a position parallel to your other leg.

10. Repeat on the other side.

Variation 2: Freestanding

This variation is similar to the first one, but without the use of a chair for balance.

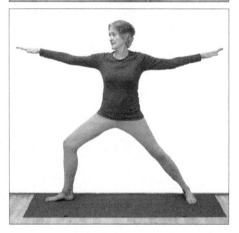

Reflections

- What is the best distance for you to have between your feet in this pose?
- How does awareness of your feet help you in this pose?
- Can you embody the confidence and strength of the warrior?

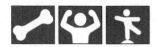

Side Angle Pose

Parsvakonasana

parsh-vah-koh-NAH-suh-nuh

Side angle pose continues from the shape of the warrior 2 pose, adding a sideways bend of the torso, which increases the bone stimulation in your lower back and hips. It also builds strength in multiple areas of the body.

Benefit: To stimulate the hip and pelvic bones while building strength, confidence and balance

Props: A yoga mat, block, chair without arms and wall (optional)

Finer Points

- If your hips feel constricted by the chair, try adding a folded blanket under your hips.
- Notice the stabilizing and expanding energies at the same time.
- As you become more confident in the mechanics of the pose, practice the expanding energies more.

Instructions

There are two variations for this pose: sitting and standing. Sitting allows you to practice the shape without having to balance, while standing helps you to build strength.

If you're just beginning, you may want to start with the sitting variation, and then progress to the standing version once you've gained more confidence.

Having a wall behind you when practicing the standing variation aids with balance until you feel more comfortable.

Variation 1: Sitting

1. Place the chair in the middle of the mat with the seat facing the long side of the mat.
2. Sit near the front edge of the chair and spread your legs apart.

3. Point your right foot and knee toward the end of the mat, with the knee over the ankle and tracking toward the second and third toes.

4. Reach your left leg to the left with your toes pointing toward the long side of the mat. If needed, adjust your position for comfort. The back knee can be bent in this variation.

5. Press down through the four corners of each foot.

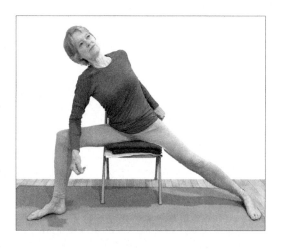

6. Lean to the right, bringing your right forearm to your thigh, pushing your right thigh toward the wall.

7. Reach your left arm behind you to touch the chair and rotate your torso toward the left.

8. Create a strong core and expand from there through your whole body.

9. Hold the pose as long as you can with strength and full awareness.

10. When you're ready, come up and rest.

11. Repeat on the other side.

Variation 2: Standing

1. Stand with your feet about 3′ apart and your back parallel to the wall for extra confidence.

2. Turn your right foot and leg out to be parallel to the long edge of your mat, leaving your left foot parallel to the short end of the mat. This will turn your pelvis slightly to the right. From the waist up, face the long edge of the mat.

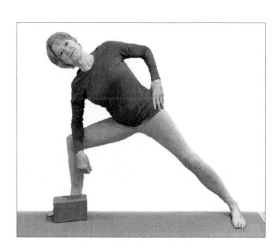

3. Place the block on the big toe side of your right foot.

4. With your upper body directly vertical over your pelvis, spread your arms wide apart.

5. Squeeze your shoulder blades toward the spine, and at the same time, stretch out through your fingers.

6. Inhaling, elongate your spine while remaining steady on your legs.

7. Exhaling, bend your right knee, bringing it directly over your ankle, pointing toward your second and third toes. This alignment is crucial to prevent straining your knee.

8. Lean your upper body to the right, bringing your forearm to your thigh and your left hand onto your hip.

9. Roll your left shoulder back.

10. Maintain strength in your extended leg, anchoring the little-toe side of your foot and contracting the thigh muscles.

11. Press down through the four corners of both feet.

12. Lengthen your tailbone toward the heel of your extended leg.

You can stay here or continue on.

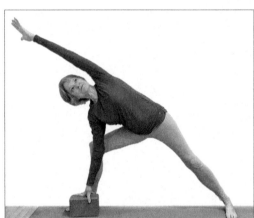

13. Bring your right hand to the block on the instep of your foot.

14. Turn your torso toward the ceiling as much as possible while looking slightly upward.

15. Stretch your left arm straight up, then alongside your head.

16. Create a strong core and expand from there through your whole body.

17. Breathe steadily as you hold the pose as long as you can.

18. When you're ready, return to standing and bring your feet together to rest.

19. Repeat on the other side.

Reflections

- What amount of support is best for you (the chair, the wall, or the block)?

- Once you are comfortable making the shape of the pose, can you energize it more?

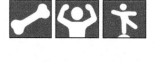

Tree Pose

Vrksasana

vrik-SHAH-suh-nuh

Tree pose is a well-known standing pose, named for the tree-like stability of one leg as your trunk and the expansion of the upper body as branches. One foot is lifted with its sole pressed against the other leg, in combination with variable arm positions.

The classic pose is done with the arms stretching straight up, possibly joining your palms, but this is not a necessary aspect of the pose. Experiment with different arm positions to find the best one for you. The goal is to be strong, expanded and able to balance without strain.

Benefit: To develop focus, balance and strength

Props: A yoga mat, chair and wall (optional)

Finer Points

- Be careful with the alignment of your standing leg and foot, as it helps your balance.
- Remember you have choices about your arm position. Try different variations.
- Experiment with the use of a chair or wall for support, building your skill and confidence gradually.

Instructions

There are three variations for this pose, each one using less support than the one before. In the first, most of your body's weight is supported by one foot while the other is resting on a chair seat. In the second, you touch a chair with your hand while standing on one leg. In the third, you balance on one foot with a wall nearby in case you need it for support.

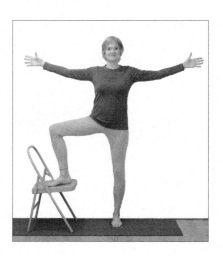

Variation 1: Foot on the chair

1. Stand on the mat with your feet parallel to each other and your back to the wall. The chair seat should be facing your right side.

2. Place your right foot on the seat, pointing your knee and foot at the same angle to the side. The exact angle will vary according to your hip structure and flexibility.

3. Press down through the four corners of the standing foot.

4. Face your pelvis straight ahead to stabilize it.

5. Focus your gaze on something straight in front of you to help you balance.

6. Inhaling, lift your arms to the sides or higher.

7. Add the expanding energy from the pelvis through your entire upper body.

8. Hold the pose for 15–30 seconds while breathing steadily.

9. When you're ready, lower your arms and bring your right foot down off the chair to stand on two feet as you rest for several breaths.

10. Move the chair to your left side and repeat the pose with your left foot on the seat.

Variation 2: One hand on the chair

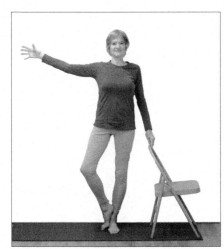

1. Stand on the mat with your feet parallel to each other and your back to the wall. The chair should be on your left side with the seat turned away from you.

2. Hold the back of the chair with your left hand.

3. Spread the toes of your left foot and press down through the four corners of that foot.

4. Lift your right foot and place its sole on the inseam of your left leg, either below or above the knee.

5. Press your foot and the standing leg into each other.

6. Contract your left thigh muscles to stabilize your knee.

7. Align your pelvis over your standing leg by moving your thighs slightly back, then lengthening your tailbone and lifting your abdomen.

8. Focus your gaze on something straight in front of you to help you balance.

9. Inhaling, raise your right arm to the side or vertically while expanding from your center.

10. Hold the pose as long as you can.

11. When you're ready, lower your right foot and arm to stand on two feet as you rest for several breaths.

12. Move the chair to your other side and repeat the pose standing on your other foot.

If you wish, you can stand with your back near a wall to give you more confidence.

Variation 3: Freestanding

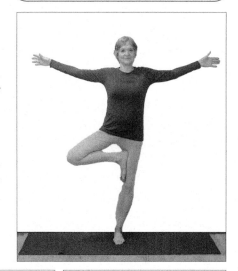

1. Stand on the mat with your feet parallel to each other and close together, spread the toes of both feet, and press down through the four corners of each foot.

2. Focus on something straight in front of you.

3. Lift your right foot, placing the sole of the foot against the inseam of your left leg, either below or above the knee.

4. Contract your left thigh muscles to stabilize your knee.

5. Align your pelvis over your standing leg by moving your thighs slightly back, then lengthening your tailbone and lifting your abdomen.

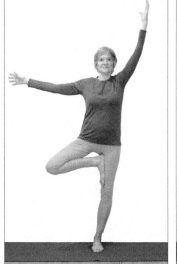

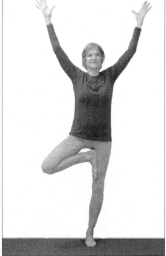

6. Inhaling, raise your arms to the side or vertically while expanding from your center, touching the wall as needed. Or, if you wish, join your hands together in front of your chest.

7. Hold the pose as long as you can.

8. When you're ready, lower your arms and stand on two feet as you rest for several breaths.

9. Repeat on the other side.

Reflections

- Can you balance more easily on one leg than the other?
- Can you feel how this pose develops sharp focus and patience?

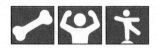

The next two poses, the triangle and half moon poses, can be done as a series once you learn them. Simply do both on the right, then both on the left.

Triangle Pose

Trikonasana

trih-koh-NAH-suh-nuh

In triangle pose, your legs remain straight and your upper body moves sideways over one leg, creating a strong stimulation to the bones of the lower back and hips, as well as presenting an opportunity to work on balance.

Benefit: To build strength, balance and coordination while stretching the outer thigh and stimulating the pelvic bones and lower back

Props: A yoga mat, block, wall and chair

Finer Points

- Your knees may want to bend, but use your intention and strength to keep them straight. This pose invites you to lengthen all the straight lines in the shape, including your legs, spine and arms.
- Use the expanding energy to help your balance.

Instructions

There are three progressive variations that increasingly challenge your balance. The distance between your feet affects your balance. A shorter stance will feel more stable, but will reduce your range of motion. A wider stance is more demanding of your flexibility, but better for bone stimulation. Find the position that feels right to you.

Variation 1: With the chair and the wall

1. Place the mat with its long edge parallel to the wall and the chair at the short edge with the seat facing you.
2. With your back to the wall, stand with your feet about 3′ apart.
3. Turn your right foot and leg out toward the end of the mat, parallel to its long edge with your toes under the chair just a bit.

4. Turn your left foot so it is parallel to the short end of the mat.

5. Press down through the four corners of each foot and retain that awareness while in the pose.

6. Ensure your upper body is parallel to the wall.

7. Activate the muscles of both legs, straightening your knees, and lift your spine up and out from the pelvis.

8. Move your sitting bones back and apart.

9. Inhaling, spread your arms wide to the sides, palms facing away from the wall.

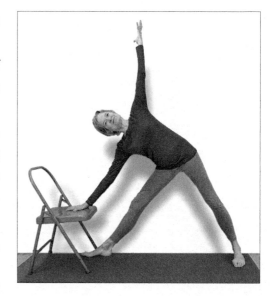

10. Exhaling, shift your hips to the left and your torso to the right, leading with your right hand and placing it on the chair seat.

11. Take a full breath.

12. Draw your tailbone in and down toward your back heel, and lift your lower abdomen. This will support your lower back and align the pelvis for good stability. It will also allow you to keep your whole body parallel to the wall rather than leaning away from the wall with your torso. This builds stronger balance.

13. With your left hand reaching toward the ceiling, roll your left shoulder and ribs up and backward as much as possible. Your spine rotates to your left. If you feel unsteady, lean lightly into the wall.

14. Expand from your pelvis out through your spine, legs and arms, with confidence and full presence.

15. Inhale as you come up, then breathe to rest.

16. Repeat on the other side.

Variation 2: With the block and the wall

1. Place the mat with its long edge parallel to the wall and the block on the floor at the short edge of the mat.

2. With your back to the wall, stand with your feet about 3′ apart.

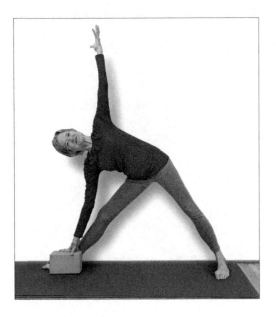

3. Turn your right foot and leg out toward the end of the mat, parallel to its long edge with your big toe beside the block. Start with the block at its highest dimension and lower it as you're ready to.

4. Turn your left foot so it is parallel to the short end of the mat.

5. Press down through the four corners of each foot and retain that awareness while in the pose.

6. Ensure your upper body is parallel to the wall.

7. Activate the muscles of both legs, straightening your knees, and lift your spine up and out from the pelvis.

8. Move your sitting bones back and apart.

9. Inhaling, spread your arms wide to the sides, palms facing away from the wall.

10. Exhaling, shift your hips to the left and your torso to the right, leading with your right hand and placing it on the block.

11. Take a full breath.

12. Draw your tailbone in and down toward your back heel, and lift your lower abdomen. This will support your lower back and align the pelvis for good stability. It will also allow you to keep your whole body parallel to the wall rather than leaning away from the wall with your torso. This builds stronger balance.

13. With your left hand reaching toward the ceiling, roll your left shoulder and ribs up and backward as much as possible. Your spine rotates to your left. If you feel unsteady, lean lightly into the wall.

14. Expand from your pelvis out through your spine, legs and arms, with confidence and full presence.

15. Inhale as you come up, then breathe to rest.

16. Repeat on the other side.

Variation 3: Freestanding with the block

The instructions for this variation are identical to the one before it, however, this time, rather than having the wall immediately behind you, imagine it there instead and position your upper body parallel to it. This is more of a psychological challenge than a physical one.

Reflections

- As you lean toward the side with your torso, can you keep your back foot grounded?
- Once you understand the biomechanics of this pose, can you expand into it more?

Half Moon Pose

Ardha Chandrasana

ar-dah chan-DRAH-suh-nuh

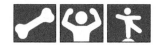

The half moon pose continues from triangle pose, since it begins with the same foundation and sideways shift of the torso. But it becomes a balance pose supported by one hand and one foot.

Benefit: To work on balance while strengthening the entire body in this side-bending shape

Props: A yoga mat, block, wall and chair

Finer Points

- One common tendency is to shift the upper body away from the wall, out of line with the pelvis and back leg. Attempt to align your body in a straight line with the wall. This gives your pelvic bones and lumbar spine a significantly more beneficial stimulation.
- Maintain the outward rotation of your standing leg, which is crucial for your balance.
- Observe both the strength and stretch that the pose offers.

Instructions

There are three variations to this pose, each using varying forms of support: a chair and the wall, a block and the wall, or freestanding.

Using the wall in the first two variations helps you to learn the shape and alignment of the pose, so I recommend using it until you are confident with your balance.

Variation 1: With a chair and the wall

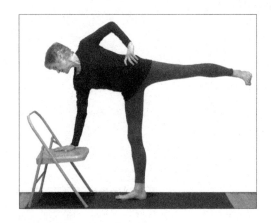

1. Place your mat parallel to the wall with a chair at the short end of the mat, its seat facing you.
2. Stand with your back to the wall and your feet about 3′ or more apart.
3. Turn your right foot and leg toward the end of the mat, parallel to its long edge, with your toes about 8–10″ in front of the chair seat. Your left foot should be parallel to the end of the mat.
4. Press down through the four corners of each foot and retain that awareness while in the pose.
5. Look toward the chair, bend your right knee, and place your right hand on the chair seat as you lift your left foot off the floor.
6. Raise the leg as high as possible and stretch it behind you, in line with your body, pointing your toes away from the wall.
7. Straighten your right knee if you're able to. Your weight is now supported by your right foot and right hand. Your right hand can move more toward the back of the seat for easier balance.
8. Place your left hand on your left hip and roll your shoulder back.
9. Check that your right knee is pointing toward the second and third toes, and use your hip muscles to retain the outward rotation of that leg. That's the key to your stability in this pose.
10. If your pelvis turns toward the floor, rotate it up toward the ceiling while maintaining the stability of your right leg.
11. If your balance is unsteady, keep your right knee slightly bent, but lift and straighten your left leg behind you. Lean against the wall with your right hip if you need support. Looking at the floor will also help you keep your balance.

12. Straighten your standing leg if you can, with the knee pointing directly toward the chair.

13. Expand from your pelvis throughout your whole body with the power of your breath.

14. Hold the pose as long as you can.

15. When you're ready, carefully return to standing on two feet and breathe to rest.

16. Prepare for the second side by moving the chair to the other end of your mat.

17. Repeat on the other side.

Variation 2: With a block

1. Place the mat with its long edge parallel to the wall and the block on the floor at the short end of the mat.

2. Stand with your back to the wall and your feet about 3′ or more apart.

3. Turn your right foot and leg toward the end of the mat, parallel to its long edge with the block about 8–10″ in front of your foot and 3″ to the right. Your left foot should be parallel to the end of the mat.

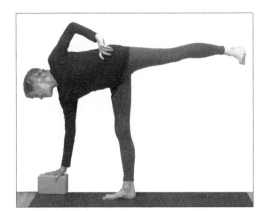

4. Press down through the four corners of each foot and retain that awareness while in the pose.

5. Look toward your right foot, bend your right knee, and place your right hand on the block as you lift your left foot off the floor.

6. Raise the leg as high as possible and stretch it behind you, in line with your body, pointing your toes away from the wall.

7. Straighten your right knee if you're able to. Your weight is now supported by your right foot and right hand.

8. Place your left hand on your left hip and roll your shoulder back.

9. Check that your right knee is pointing toward the second and third toes, and use your hip muscles to retain the

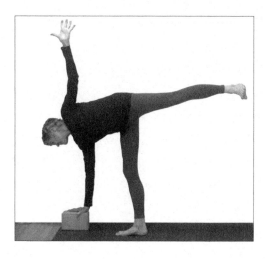

outward rotation of that leg. That's the key to your stability in this pose.

10. If your pelvis turns toward the floor, rotate it up toward the ceiling while maintaining the stability of your right leg.

11. If your balance is unsteady, keep your right knee slightly bent, but lift and straighten your left leg behind you. Lean against the wall with your right hip if you need support. Looking at the floor will also help you keep your balance.

12. Straighten your standing leg if you can.

13. Expand from your pelvis throughout your whole body with the power of your breath.

14. Hold the pose as long as you can.

15. When you're ready, carefully return to standing on two feet and breathe to rest.

16. Prepare for the second side by moving the block to the other end of your mat.

17. Repeat on the other side.

Variation 3: Freestanding with a block

The instructions for this variation are similar to the one before it, however, this time, rather than having the wall immediately behind you, imagine it there instead and position your upper body parallel to it. This is more of a psychological challenge than a physical one. To increase its benefits, raise your left hand in the air to expand the pose.

Reflections

- Once you understand the biomechanics of this pose, can you expand into it more?
- How does it feel different from other balancing poses?

One-Legged Standing Twist

In this standing twist, one foot is on the chair as you stabilize your pelvis and turn your upper body. It's a variation of a seated

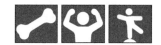

pose, adding the element of balance to the twist and preparing you for similar poses to come.

Benefit: To practice focus and balance while stimulating the pelvic bones and lumbar spine

Props: A yoga mat and chair

Finer Points

- One common tendency is to lean heavily into the chair. To prevent that, align your standing leg vertically with your hips over your ankles. Most of your weight should be on your standing leg.

- When twisting to the right, your left leg, hip and side will tend to move forward into the twist. Resist that by pulling the left hip and thigh (the side you're turning away from) back slightly. Another way to keep the pelvis steady and facing the chair is to guide your right hip gently forward with your right hand.

Instructions

1. Place a chair at the short end of the mat, with the front of the seat toward you.

2. Face the chair seat and stand tall in mountain pose. (If needed, you can review this pose on page 59.)

3. Lift your right foot onto the chair seat, pointing your pelvis and right knee straight ahead.

4. Straighten your left leg and lift your spine up and out of the pelvis.

5. Reach your sitting bones back and apart, which will arch your lower spine slightly.

6. Lengthen your tailbone and lift your lower abdomen, coming to a neutral pelvic tilt to stabilize your torso over your standing leg.

7. Place your left hand on your right knee, and your right hand on your hip.

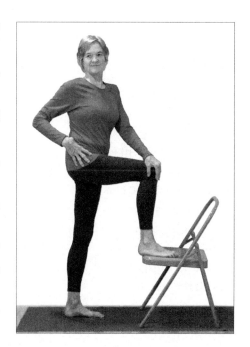

8. Inhale while you stretch up and turn your upper torso to the right. If you're feeling unstable, pull your left thigh back.

9. Squeeze your shoulder blades toward the spine and away from your ears.

10. Exhale while you turn your ribs, shoulders and head, focusing on something on the horizon to help you balance. Avoid letting your pelvis turn.

11. Broaden your chest with each inhale, and as you exhale, continue to empower the twist from your spine, ribs and abdomen.

12. Hold as long as you can.

13. When you're ready, release the twist and return your foot to the floor while breathing to rest.

14. Repeat on the other side.

Reflections

- As you turn your upper body to one side, can you keep your pelvis facing the chair?
- How far can you twist your upper body without moving your pelvis?

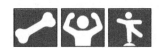

The standing variations of the next two poses, warrior 1 and warrior 3, can be done as a series once you learn them. First do both poses on the right, then both on the left.

Warrior 1

Virabhadrasana 1

vee-rah-bah-DRAH-suh-nuh

Warrior 1 pose energizes the whole body and mind as you become the yogic warrior. With one leg forward and one leg back, you maintain a steady pelvis. This shape utilizes precise alignment and requires sharp mental focus to maintain balance.

Benefit: To build strength, develop balance, and stimulate the bones of the pelvis and spine

Props: A yoga mat, chair without arms, small pad and blanket or block (optional)

Finer Points

- Carefully align your pelvis to face the end of your mat, adjusting your feet as needed.

- As you lift your torso into the backbend, notice the stretch and strength required.
- Take care to establish your balance before releasing your hands from the chair.

Instructions

There are two variations of this pose: sitting and standing. The sitting version gives you an accessible starting point and allows you to refine your alignment, while the standing version helps to develop balance and strength.

You can use a folded blanket or block for height adjustments in the sitting variation as needed. If you are tall, place a folded blanket under you on the chair. If you are short, position a block or folded blanket under your front foot.

Variation 1: Sitting

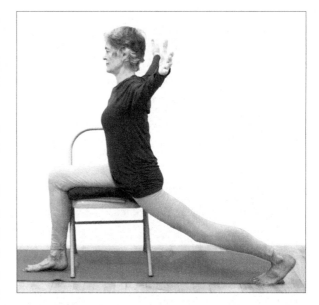

1. Place a chair in the middle of your mat, with the seat facing its long edge.
2. Sit sideways in the chair with your right thigh along its front edge, so your left hip is off the seat.
3. Extend your left leg about 3′ behind you, pressing your toes into the mat and lifting your heel.
4. Point your right knee, right foot and both sides of your pelvis toward the short end of the mat. When the left leg stretches back, it may pull your pelvis to that side. So you may need to rotate your pelvis to the right to face straight ahead again.
5. Hold the chair if needed while you lean forward slightly and reach your sitting bones back and apart. Then lengthen your tailbone and lift your lower abdomen. These movements will help stabilize your pelvis for the next stage of the pose.

6. Maintain these actions as you bring your head and shoulders back over your pelvis. You'll notice the front of your left hip stretching.

7. Lift your spine and bring your arms out to the sides. Press into the floor as if you were about to lift off the chair, preparing for the next stage.

8. Hold the pose as long as you can, breathing steadily and maintaining the expanding energy.

9. When you're ready, bring the back leg forward and turn to sit comfortably in the chair.

10. Repeat on the other side.

Variation 2: Standing

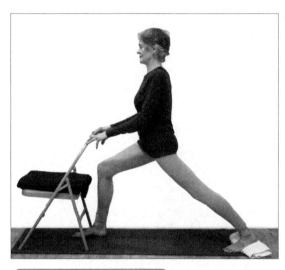

Use a small pad (like a folded towel or second yoga mat) to support your heel at the back of the mat.

1. Place a chair at the short end of the mat, with the back of the chair facing you.

2. Hold the chair back lightly for balance while stepping your right foot forward until your toes are just under the chair.

3. Bend your right knee, pointing it toward the second and third toes.

4. Extend your left leg about 3′ behind you, turning it out slightly and placing your heel on the small pad you placed there.

5. Leaning forward slightly, check that your pelvis is evenly facing the chair, not turned toward the back leg.

6. Create the anterior tilt of your pelvis, reaching back and apart with your sitting bones and upper thighs.

7. Lengthen your tailbone and lift your lower abdomen to create stability in your pelvis and lower back.

8. Bring your torso upright as you lift your spine.

9. Squeeze your shoulder blades toward each other.

10. Establish your balance, looking straight ahead and touching the chair very lightly.

11. If and when you are ready, stretch one or both arms to the sides.

12. If you are steady enough to do so, try to lift one or both arms next to your head or as high as they will go.

13. Breathe fully.

To increase the challenge of this pose:

14. Arch your upper back and look up, performing a neck extension (as shown on page 54).

15. Stretch your back leg more vigorously.

16. Expand energetically in all directions from your center.

17. When you're ready, release the pose and breathe deeply as you rest.

18. Repeat on the other side.

Reflections

• Can you remain aware of your alignment, balance, strength and breathing all at once in this pose?

• Can you feel the warrior qualities of strength and courage in this pose?

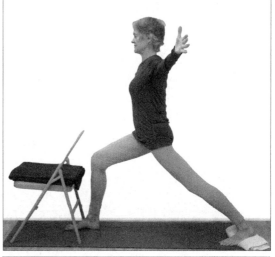

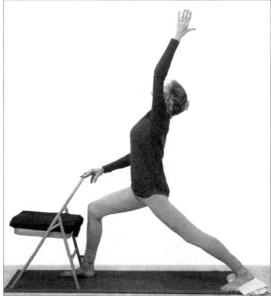

Variation 2 can be the entry into the next pose, warrior 3. When doing this sequence, step away from the chair about 8–12″ before transitioning from warrior 1 to warrior 3.

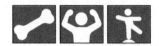

Warrior 3

Virabhadrasana 3

vee-rah-bah-DRAH-suh-nuh

Following from warrior 1, you embody that strength and courage in a one-legged stance. The shape is similar to the balancing table pose (on page 83) with one leg and the opposite arm stretching away from your center. However, this pose is done standing on one leg, instead of being on your hands and knees.

Benefit: To increase strength and improve balance

Props: A yoga mat, chair and blanket (optional)

Finer Points

- Be sure to begin with your pelvis and standing leg facing forward, toward the chair and the end of the mat.
- Continue breathing and expand from the center of your body through your spine, arms and legs while keeping both sides of your torso long.

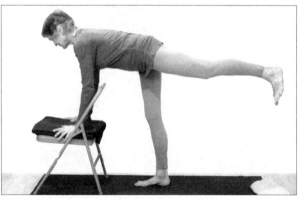

Instructions

1. Place a chair at the short end of the mat, with the seat facing away from you, and a folded blanket on it for comfort.
2. Touching the back of the chair, place your feet about 8–12″ away from it.
3. Bring your weight to your right foot and reach over the back of the chair to place your hands on the seat.
4. Lift the left leg behind you without turning your pelvis. Your navel, extended leg and toes should face downward.
5. Expand from your center with full strength.
6. Raise your right arm, stretching it forward. Feel how your right arm and your left leg balance each other across the diagonal of your body.

7. Maintain the alignment of your body facing downward and keep your abdomen strong. Hold this pose for as long as you can.

8. When you're ready, return to standing upright on two feet and rest.

9. Repeat on the other side.

Reflections

- Can you expand with enthusiasm in this pose?
- Does this pose remind you of the balancing table pose?

Revolved Triangle Pose

Parivrtta Trikonasana

pah-ree-vrih-tah trih-koh-NAH-suh-nuh

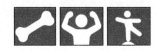

In revolved triangle pose, your legs are separated with one in front and one behind, and your upper body tilts forward and twists over the front leg. It is a strong stretch for your leading hip and a good strengthener for your spine and abdomen.

Benefit: To strengthen the legs and spine (both bones and muscles), stimulate the vertebrae with twisting, and improve balance

Props: A yoga mat, chair and one or two blocks (optional)

These next two poses, revolved triangle and revolved side angle, both involve strong twists. At first, choose just one or the other to include in your practice on any given day. Include both when you're confident about each pose.

Finer Points

- Prioritize alignment over range of motion. Stabilizing your pelvis is more important than how far you twist.
- To help you balance, inch your feet a bit farther away from the midline. Experiment to find the best width for you.
- As you remain in the pose, inhale to elongate and exhale to twist.

Instructions

There are two variations: one with a chair and the other with a block. The chair variation requires less flexibility and balance, while the block variation helps develop strength and stamina.

Variation 1: With a chair

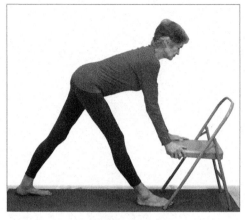

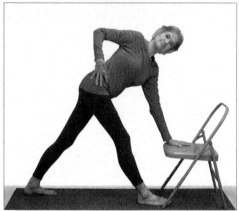

1. Place a chair at the short end of the mat, with the front of the seat toward you.
2. Stand facing the chair about 2–3′ away with your legs parallel to each other. Take special care to align both sides of your pelvis evenly toward the end of the mat.
3. Bend forward at your hips, placing both hands on the seat.
4. Elongate your spine and legs. This is hip flexion without spin al flexion.
5. Step forward with your right foot, bringing your toes under the front of the chair.
6. Turn your left leg out slightly, so the toes are pointing to eleven on an imaginary clock face. In doing so, keep your pelvis square to the chair, which may require shifting your navel slightly to the right.
7. Press down through the four corners of your feet for good support.
8. Take another breath to elongate your spine again.
9. As you exhale, turn your torso (from your navel upward) to the right, leaving your left hand on the chair seat, and place your right hand on your hip. Roll that shoulder back.
10. Notice how your pelvis wants to turn as well. Restrain it by pushing into the outer heel of your back foot.
11. Stretch both legs and your spine fully, elongating through your sitting bones as well as your spine and head.
12. Hold as long as possible, breathing steadily.
13. When you're ready, release the pose, then return to standing upright with both feet together and rest.
14. Repeat on the other side.

Variation 2: With a block

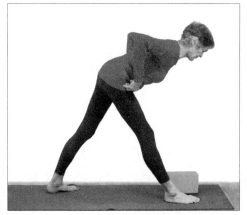

1. Place a block at the short end of the mat on the left side.
2. Step forward with your right foot, placing it parallel to the block, which should be about 1′ to the left.
3. Move your left leg about 3′ back.
4. Turn your left leg out slightly, so the toes are pointing to eleven on an imaginary clock face. In doing so, keep your pelvis square to the end of the mat, which may require shifting your navel slightly to the right.
5. Press down through the four corners of your feet for good support.
6. Bend forward at your hips, keeping your spine long.

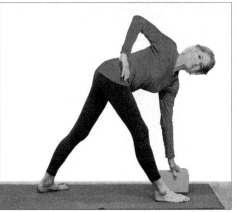

7. Place your left hand on the block.
8. Take another breath to elongate your spine again.
9. As you exhale, turn your torso (from your navel upward) to the right and place your right hand on your hip.
10. Roll that shoulder back. Notice how your pelvis wants to turn as well. Restrain it by pushing into the outer heel of your back foot.
11. Stretch both legs and your spine fully, elongating through your sitting bones as well as your spine and head.
12. Hold as long as possible, breathing steadily.
13. When you're ready, release the pose, then return to standing upright with both feet together and rest.
14. Repeat on the other side.

Reflections

- What parts of your body are working strongly in this pose?
- Can you maintain a steady breathing rhythm while twisting?

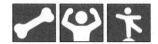

Revolved Side Angle Pose

Parivrtta Parsvakonasana

pah-ree-vrih-tah parsh-vah-koh-NAH-suh-nuh

Revolved side angle pose is another standing twist, but this time with your front leg bent. Working with a chair will help you to remain well aligned as you twist your spine.

Benefit: To strengthen the legs and spine, stimulate the vertebrae and the vertebral muscles, and improve balance

Props: A yoga mat, chair without arms and blanket or block (optional)

Finer Points

- Prioritize alignment and stability more than range of motion in the twist.
- Avoid forcing the twist with your arms.
- Note the tendency to lean your upper body toward the back of the chair. Instead, align your head with your back foot.
- Increase all the actions to lift your pelvis off the chair.

> You can use a folded blanket or block for height adjustments as needed. If you are tall, place a folded blanket under you on the chair. If you are short, position a block or folded blanket under your front foot.

Instructions

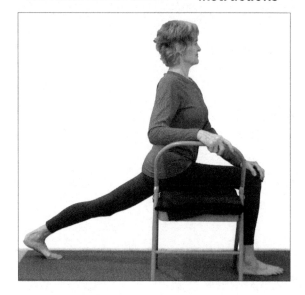

1. Place the chair next to the mat at its center with the seat facing the long edge. It's best if the two back legs of the chair are off the mat.
2. Set the folded blanket on the seat, depending on your height and flexibility.
3. Sit sideways in the chair, facing to the right, with your right thigh along the front edge of the chair, so your left hip is off the seat.
4. Stretch your left foot behind you, pressing your toes into the mat and lifting your heel, with your knee bent slightly.
5. Point your right knee, right foot and both sides of your pelvis toward the short end of the mat. When the left leg stretches back,

it may pull your pelvis to that side. So you may need to rotate your pelvis to the right to face straight ahead again.

6. Lean forward and extend your back leg.

7. Reach your sitting bones back and apart, which will arch your lower spine slightly.

8. Lengthen your tailbone and lift your abdomen, coming to a neutral pelvic tilt.

9. Stretch your back leg as much as you can.

10. Inhale as you lengthen your spine up and out of the pelvis.

11. Exhale and turn your torso to the right, holding the chair with both hands. Your torso is angling forward, but not collapsing toward the front leg.

12. Keep your shoulders broad and your head in line with your pelvis.

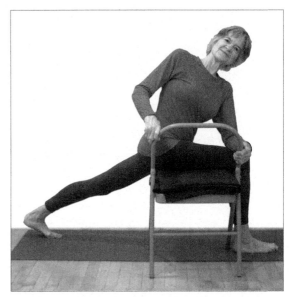

13. Hold the pose, elongating as you inhale and twisting more as you exhale.

14. If you wish, lift your pelvis off the chair while maintaining the shape to give your bones and muscles more stimulation.

15. When you're ready, release the pose and rest.

16. To repeat on the other side, sit with your left side toward the back of the chair.

Reflections

- How does the chair help you in this pose?
- Can you feel the strong center in your pelvis, with the one leg stretching back and your spine tilting forward as you twist?

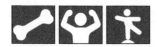

Wide-Legged Standing Forward Bend

Prasarita Padottanasana

prah-SAH-rih-tah pah-doh-tah-NAH-suh-nuh

The wide-legged standing forward bend is a symmetrical pose that provides a good way to finish your active practice and transition toward relaxation. You'll rest your head in a gentle forward-folded position, while your feet are spread apart.

Benefit: To stretch your hips and thighs, stimulate the bones of your pelvis and spine, and calm your mind and your breathing

Props: A mat, chair, blanket and one or two blocks

Finer Points

- This is a forward bend, so take care to elongate your spine, allowing only a small amount of curvature as you fold forward with your upper body.
- If your legs are stiff, you can bend your knees at first to find an anterior tilt of your pelvis and to lengthen your spine. Gradually work to straighten your legs.
- Maintain active strength in your legs as you soften your upper body into the support of the chair or blocks.
- Adjust the height of your support (blankets or blocks on the chair seat) using as much as you need to rest your head comfortably without rounding your spine.

Instructions

This pose is intentionally the last standing pose because it is calming after a strenuous practice.

1. Place the chair next to the mat at its center with the seat facing the long edge. It's best if the two back legs of the chair are off the mat.
2. Set the folded blanket and one block (or more) on the seat, depending on your height and flexibility.
3. Stand facing the chair with your legs 3–4' apart, your feet parallel, and the four corners of each foot pressing into the floor.
4. Inhaling, extend your legs and elongate your spine up and out of the pelvis.

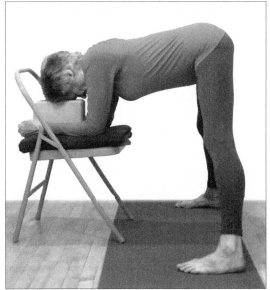

5. Exhaling, bend forward by folding at the hips (not the spine) and bring your hands to the chair seat. Your arms are straight to begin with and your torso is roughly parallel to the floor.

6. Reach your sitting bones back and apart and keep your hips above your ankles.

7. Practice the stabilizing and expanding energies. From a strong core in the center of your body, press down through your legs and up through your spine and head.

8. See if you can bend forward more to rest your forearms on the chair and your head on the block without rounding your spine. The limiting factor here is hip mobility, so be self-aware and don't force it. You can put another folded blanket on the seat to make it higher if needed.

9. Rest your head on the block and adjust its position for neck comfort.

10. Once your head is supported, bring your attention to your breathing. Guide it to become more smooth, slow and steady, while quieting your mind.

11. Remain in the pose as long as you wish.

12. When you're ready, straighten your arms to come out of the pose the same way you went in. Step closer to the chair and bend your knees as you stand.

Reflections

- Can you bend forward from your hips more at the end of the practice than you could at the beginning?
- Can you acknowledge your efforts with self-appreciation?

Chapter 12. **Cool-down Series**

The poses in the cool-down series allow you time to rest after physical exertion, to assimilate your gains, and to quiet your mind. Dress appropriately for the room temperature and reduce any distractions as you rest. You can practice all three poses at the end of a yoga session or choose just one or two.

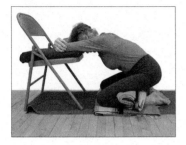

Child's Pose

Balasana

bah-LAH-suh-nuh

Child's pose is a well-known resting yoga pose. In these variations, we use extra props to ensure safe spinal alignment and protection from possible discomfort in the knees as we rest the spine.

For complete instructions on how to do this pose, refer to "Child's Pose" on page 94.

Corpse Pose with Legs on a Chair

Savasana (or Shavasana)

shah-VAH-suh-nuh

This variation of corpse pose is done with a folded blanket under your spine and your lower legs on the seat of a chair. Resting quietly with your legs elevated allows your mind and body to relax deeply.

Benefit: To relieve fatigue and reduce stress

Props: A yoga mat, chair, two to four blankets and towel (optional)

Finer Points

- Using a long narrow blanket under your spine (but not your pelvis) will create a slight anterior tilt. Check for that.
- Connect with your breath, allowing it to deepen and slow down. Prolong your exhalation.

Instructions

1. Place a chair at the short end of your mat with the seat either facing you or to the side. Depending on the design of your chair and the length of your legs, a sideways position may work better.
2. Set a folded blanket on the seat for comfort.
3. Fold a second blanket into a long and narrow shape, which will cushion your spine. Place it on the mat about 6–8˝ away from the front of the chair.

4. Facing to the side, sit on the mat between the blanket and the chair.

5. Lie down on the blanket by pivoting on your hips, then lift your lower legs onto the seat. You may need to adjust the position of the chair to fully support your calves. Adding another blanket over you (or a purring cat!) will help you relax.

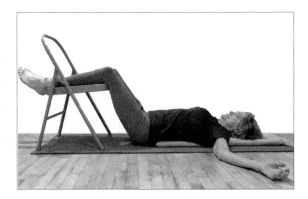

6. For a bit more comfort, you can add a folded towel or blanket under your neck and head.

7. If you feel any compression in your lower back, lengthen your tailbone toward the chair.

8. Rest your arms out to the sides with your palms facing up.

9. Gently shift your shoulder blades toward your spine and relax your neck and face.

10. Guide your awareness throughout your whole body, letting each part relax and receive the support of the floor and props as much as possible.

11. Let your mind and body relax together. As you notice thoughts arising, witness them without getting involved. Bring your attention back to your breath. Be patient and loving toward yourself.

12. After resting for 5–10 minutes, gently deepen your inhalation, which will wake you up more, and move in any way that feels right.

13. When you're ready, take your legs off the chair and come up to a sitting position.

14. Reflect on your experience of the practice and affirm your commitment to your well-being on every level.

Reflections

- What physical sensations arise as you rest?
- What thoughts go through your mind as you reflect on your practice?
- Can you let your thoughts come and go without being pulled into them?

Mountain Brook

Savasana (or Shavasana)

shah-VAH-suh-nuh

Mountain brook is another variation of corpse pose, which supports the contours of the body as it releases, becoming soft and fluid like water flowing over stones in a brook. Your spine and shoulders will relax, and your breathing will soften and expand.

Benefit: To relax and absorb the benefits of your practice

Props: A yoga mat, two blankets, a bolster and an eye mask (optional)

Finer Points

- Make any adjustments you need for comfort.

Instructions

1. Arrange the two blankets on the mat so you have a rolled one for your neck and head and a folded one for your mid-back where its upper edge should be just touching the base of your shoulder blades. The bolster will support your knees.

2. Lie down on the mat and adjust the blankets as needed. Be sure that the middle one is gently lifting your chest, and that your shoulders are on the mat, not on a blanket.

3. If you feel any compression in your lower back, lengthen your pelvis toward your legs.

4. Cover your eyes to block the light if you wish.

5. Rest your arms out to the sides with your palms facing up.

6. Gently shift your shoulder blades toward your spine.

7. Guide your awareness throughout your whole body, letting each part relax and receive the support of the floor and props as much as possible.

8. Let your mind and body relax together. As you notice thoughts arising, witness them without getting involved. Bring your attention back to your breath. Be patient and loving toward yourself.

9. After resting for 5–10 minutes, gently deepen your inhalation, which will wake you up more, and move in any way that feels right.

10. When you're ready, come up to a sitting position.

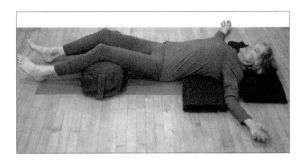

Reflect on your experience of the practice and affirm your commitment to your well-being on every level.

> Congratulations!
> You're done!
> Enjoy the fruits of your practice!

Parting Thoughts

In *Empowered Aging*, my purpose has been to encourage you to develop and maintain a safe and enjoyable practice of yoga to be vibrantly active in your elder years. Some form of exercise is essential for both our general fitness and mental health, but especially to keep our muscles and bones as strong as possible. But what kind of exercise? Many popular sports or gym workouts might be risky if you have arthritis, low bone density, weak muscles, cardiovascular issues, or other health conditions.

Yoga is adaptable for people with any level of experience, flexibility, strength and coordination. You can start gently and build up little by little. The warm-up sequences included in this book will help you ease into the practice while gaining confidence and skill, and you can use props to reduce the challenge of poses as you learn them. This book provides plenty of options.

Although our bones tend to lose density and become more prone to fracture as we age, we can proactively slow that process by giving our bones appropriate stimulation as part of our yoga routine. Our bones are alive, and they get stronger as we carry the weight of the body in varying positions and movements that target those areas most at risk for fracture: the spine, hips and wrists.

It's common (and frustrating) to become less confident in our stability as we get older. We might walk more slowly, feel unsteady, and lose the ability to stay in touch with the body in the movements of daily life. Balance is a body/mind skill requiring mental focus and good awareness. The yoga I've presented in this book puts a significant emphasis on being fully present with what you're doing, rather than doing it mechanically or mindlessly. And to avoid falling, we need to practice balance in a variety of ways. Be creative and include both static and dynamic exercises. The standing poses and core strength practices in this book are particularly good for improving your stability.

From a wider perspective, yoga is an integrative practice that engages your mind and body in synergy together. The attention you give to your body and sensations will carry through into better self-care during your daily life. You start to notice how feeling stronger gives you more freedom. Each skill you build through your yoga practice will serve you in any activity you choose to do.

As you incorporate practices from this book into your daily routine, I hope you will feel empowered to develop and maintain a vibrantly active life, even with the challenges of aging that we all face. Where you are right now is the best place to start. Focusing on gradually building your strength and working on your balance, while not expecting perfection, is incredibly valuable. It's a challenge to see beyond any limiting self-judgments and fears, but you can do it!

This yoga methodology, honed over many years, has shown you the specifics of optimal alignment and posture that will be an invaluable underpinning to your health in general and your yoga practice in particular. I've shared not only what poses to do, but why and how to do them. I've explained how the "inner pose," the subtle internal actions, brings the practice to life, so you're not just making shapes or imitating a photograph. Students frequently tell me what a difference it makes to experience their body in this new way. The details may be daunting at first, but will gradually become familiar and clearly beneficial, even transformational.

As you progress along the path, you will be supported by a new level of self-awareness and a sense of agency to create and maintain a workable program for yourself. If you follow the instructions in *Empowered Aging*, you'll be able to exercise safely and effectively and to see the benefits gradually increasing. Every small success gives you more enthusiasm for the next steps in your journey.

But don't feel like you have to go it alone. I welcome you to contact me and share what you're learning. You can also visit my YouTube channel (ellensaltonstall.com/youtube) for the free classes I offer there to inspire you on your journey.

May yoga be a boon to your life, bringing you optimal health and fulfillment.

Thank you for reading *Empowered Aging*.
If you've enjoyed reading this book, please leave a
review on your favorite review site. It helps me reach
more readers who may benefit from the information
provided here.

Acknowledgments

I started practicing yoga in my twenties for its health benefits, especially the way it encourages integration of the body, mind and spirit. Since that time, I have had help from many people along my path to becoming a devoted practitioner, teacher and a writer. The material in this book is the product of my most recent fifteen years of focus on how yoga can help us remain active and vibrant in our lives as we age. Over this time, I've gained wisdom from my own aging experience as well as my formal yoga training and teaching. I thank my loyal yoga students and clients for supporting me, challenging me, and fueling me to continue learning.

I have been fortunate to have studied with many brilliant teachers in the Iyengar and Anusara yoga traditions, who have provided me with a strong foundation in yoga technique, philosophy and how to craft a skillful practice. They also conveyed by example the joy of being in it long term, with all its highs and lows. In particular, I want to thank Suzanne Hodges, Mary Dunn, Judith Lasater, John Friend and Carrie Owerko. I am deeply grateful to my colleagues Barrie Risman, Nina Zolotow, Angela Caplan, Jacki McCausland, Jayendra Hanley, Jim and Ruthie Bernhaert, Susan Genis and David Fink for our lively discussions about the nuances of teaching yoga. I'm also grateful to Nina Zolotow for including me as a writer for her blog, *Yoga for Healthy Aging*. My anatomical studies with Thomas Myers and Robert Schleip have greatly enriched my understanding of the body—another never-ending field of study.

I thank Loren Fishman for our collaboration on two earlier books: *Yoga for Arthritis* (2008) and *Yoga for Osteoporosis* (2010).

The wonderful people at YogaUOnline have supported me as we continue to produce programs together, many of them about how yoga can help people with a diagnosis of osteoporosis. I thank Eva Nordlyk Smith, Lynn Crimando and Patti Hamilton for our ongoing collaborations.

I am deeply thankful to Gurumayi Chidvilasananda and my spiritual community in Siddha Yoga for inspiration and sustenance through many phases of my life and work.

For the photographs included here, I thank my family members Josef Kushner, Lynn Saltonstall, and Max Saltonstall, whose sharp eyes and good cheer helped tremendously.

Thanks also to medical illustrator Emily Ciosek, who skillfully depicts many of the concepts in the introductory chapters of this book.

Thanks to Liz Riviere for her expert help with all my digital advertising and promotion. She has guided me to be more adept at this aspect of my profession with creativity and grace.

I thank Miriam Seidel whose editorial skills helped me to create the overall form and content of this book in its first phase.

For further development, I thank Tara Alemany and Mark Gerber of Emerald Lake Books. Tara expertly guided me in editing the structure and the text with meticulous attention to detail, even as she continuously brought us back to the overall goal of this book. Mark Gerber provided excellent art direction and design, and has been a pleasure to work with.

Special thanks to my family for their ongoing support and encouragement throughout the process of producing this book.

About the Author

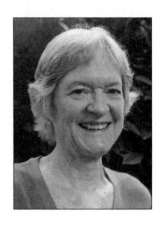

Ellen Saltonstall is an experienced yoga instructor with forty-five years of study, practice and teaching. She is known for her clarity, depth of knowledge, and enthusiasm for encouraging students of all levels to find freedom and joy through yoga.

This body of experience, passion and knowledge is the subject of Ellen's newest book, *Empowered Aging: Everyday Yoga Practices for Bone Health, Strength and Balance.* This book guides readers through her unique methodology for older students who are coming to yoga for help with the common conditions of aging.

Her certifications include an Experienced Registered Yoga Teacher (E-RYT 500) designation from the Yoga Alliance and a yoga therapist certification (C-IYAT) with the International Association of Yoga Therapists. Ellen's training is in both Iyengar yoga and Anusara yoga, and she has studied with many master teachers over the years to whom she is grateful.

Ellen holds a bachelor's degree from Cornell University and a master's degree from New York University. Her background includes studying and performing modern dance, working as a massage therapist, and appearing in two feature films: *Hair* (1978) and *Yogawoman* (2011).

She has taught at Bard College, Cornell University, and Sarah Lawrence College, instructing students in human anatomy, yoga therapeutics, and Bodymind Ballwork, a method of bodywork she developed that uses rubber balls of various sizes and textures to massage and realign the body, refine proprioception, and facilitate tension release. She explains the technique in her book, *The Bodymind Ballwork Method* (North Atlantic Books, 2018).

Ellen teaches regularly with the highly regarded online platform YogaUOnline, as well as in yoga venues both nationally and internationally, and her writings have appeared in *Yoga Journal*, *Topics in Geriatric Rehabilitation*, and The International Association of Yoga Therapists's *Journal of Yoga Therapy*.

Her other published books include *Yoga for Arthritis* (Norton, 2008) and *Yoga for Osteoporosis* (Norton, 2010), both coauthored with Dr. Loren Fishman, and *Anatomy and Yoga* (Abhyasa Press, 2016).

Ellen is based in New York City, where she maintains her yoga studio and where she and her husband, Robert Kushner, raised three wonderful human beings. For more information about the current in-person and virtual classes and workshops she is offering, visit her website at ellensaltonstall.com.

If you're interested in having Ellen speak to your group or organization or to present a workshop for you, you can contact her at emeraldlakebooks.com/saltonstall.

Recommended Resources

Anatomy and Yoga: A Guide for Teachers and Students by Ellen Saltonstall. (Abhyasa Press, 2016.) An experiential tour of the anatomical body relative to yoga practice.

Breath: The New Science of a Lost Art by James Nestor. (Penguin Random House, 2020.) A journalist's adventure-filled exploration of breathwork.

Evolving Your Yoga: Ten Principles for Enlightened Practices by Barrie Risman. (Barrie Risman, 2019.) An accessible and authentic exploration of the core teachings of yoga and how to apply them to yoga and daily life.

Enlighten Up!: Finding Clarity, Contentment and Resilience in a Complicated World by Beth Gibbs. (Emerald Lake Books, 2021.) An insightful look at contemporary life framed by the lens of a 3,000-year-old yogic teaching about the five layers of our being.

From the Boxing Ring to the Ashram: Wisdom for Mind, Body and Spirit by Deborah Charnes. (Emerald Lake Books, 2023.) A collection of engaging stories of the author's experiences while learning about the mind, body and spirit from a variety of teachers.

Light on Pranayama: The Yogic Art of Breathing by B. K. S. Iyengar. (Harper Collins, 1993.) A primer on pranayama by a yoga luminary.

Living Your Yoga: Finding the Spiritual in Everyday Life by Judith Lasater. (Rodmell Press, 2000.) An inspiring book on integrating ancient wisdom into our daily lives.

Mayo Clinic on Osteoporosis: Keep Your Bones Strong and Reduce Your Risk of Fracture by Ann E. Kearns, MD, PhD. (Mayo Clinic Press, 2021.) An excellent source of information about all aspects of osteoporosis.

Meditation for the Love of It: Enjoying Your Own Deepest Experience by Sally Kempton. (Sounds True, 2011.) An engaging, informative and personal invitation into the practice of meditation.

Outlive: The Science & Art of Longevity by Peter Attia with Bill Clifford. (Vermillion, 2023.) A compelling callout written by a physician and a medical journalist advocating for better prevention of the most common chronic diseases offering the goal of a long, resilient "healthspan." (Spoiler alert: He calls exercise the most powerful longevity drug.)

The Bodymind Ballwork Method: A Self-Directed Practice to Help you Move with Ease, Release Tension, and Relieve Chronic Pain by Ellen Saltonstall. (North Atlantic Books, 2018.) A discussion of body/mind connections, plus practical techniques for tension release.

The Breathing Book: Good Health and Vitality Through Essential Breath Work by Donna Fahri. (Henry Holt and Company, 1996.) An excellent guide to healing breathing practices for beginners.

The Deeper Dimension of Yoga: Theory and Practice by Georg Feuerstein. (Shambhala Publications, 2003.) A comprehensive and readable survey of yoga practices by one of the foremost yoga writers and historians of the twentieth century.

The Pain Management Workbook: Powerful CBT and Mindfulness Skills to Take Control of Pain and Reclaim Your Life by Rachel Zoffness. (New Harbinger Publications, 2020.) Step-by-step guidance for developing strategies to understand, manage and reduce pain.

The Principles and Practice of Yoga in Health Care by Sat Bir Singh Khalsa, Lorenzo Cohen, Timothy McCall, and Shirley Telles. eds. (Handspring Publishing, 2016.) An overview of the efficacy of yoga for medical conditions, written by a team of leading researchers.

The Yoga of Breath: A Step-by-Step Guide to Pranayama by Richard Rosen. (Shambhala Publications, 2002.) An accessible instruction book for yogic breathing practices.

The Yoga Tradition: Its History, Literature, Philosophy and Practice by Georg Feuerstein. (Hohm Press, 2001.) A comprehensive resource about all aspects of yoga, written by one of the foremost yoga writers and historians of the twentieth century.

Yoga and Scoliosis: A Journey to Health and Healing by Marcia Monroe. (DemosHealth, 2012.) A valuable resource to help those with spinal asymmetries develop a personal practice of yoga.

Yoga as Medicine: The Yogic Prescription for Health and Healing by Timothy McCall, MD. (Bantam Dell, 2007.) A guide for treating common conditions with yoga, featuring chapters by master yoga teachers.

Yoga Body: The Origins of Modern Postural Practice by Mark Singleton. (Oxford University Press, 2010.) A scholar's thoroughly researched book about the influence of twentieth-century gymnastics and bodybuilding in the development of many contemporary yoga practices.

Yoga for Arthritis: The Complete Guide by Loren Fishman and Ellen Saltonstall. (W. W. Norton, 2008.) A valuable yoga-specific resource for those with osteoarthritis who want to improve their pain-free range of movement.

Yoga for Healthy Aging: A Guide to Lifelong Well-Being by Baxter Bell, MD, and Nina Zolotow. (Shambhala Publications, 2017.) An excellent and comprehensive resource about aging and the benefits of yoga for the mind and body, from two accomplished writers and teachers of yoga.

Yoga for Osteoporosis: The Complete Guide by Loren Fishman and Ellen Saltonstall. (W. W. Norton, 2010.) A comprehensive guide for the management and prevention of osteoporosis with yoga.

Yoga for Scoliosis: A Path for Students and Teachers by Elise Browning Miller and nancy DL heraty. (nancy heraty, 2016.) A reputable guide to yoga practices for those with scoliosis.

Index

For more great books, please visit us at
emeraldlakebooks.com.

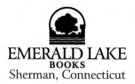

Printed in Great Britain
by Amazon

61019021R00114